Therefore in medicine we ought to know the causes of sickness and health.

Avicenna

(980 AD)

DEDICATION

TO

THE FUTURE DOCTOR

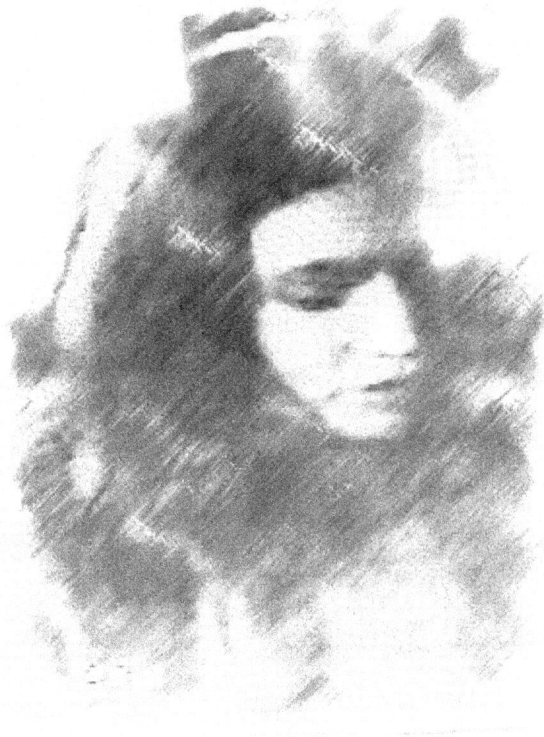

PREFACE

Getting accepted and enrolling in a medical school is one of the great adventures of life. It truly challenges one on an emotional, physical and intellectual level.

This journey is marked by tests of knowledge and skill at points along the way.

One of the first challenges in a medical student's career is the test for proficiency in the basic sciences. In the United States, it is called USMLE Step 1, in the commonwealth, it is called MBBS I and is known by other equivalents in other countries.

The key to success in exams is the ability to cover a large breadth of information in the final review period before an exam. A notebook that has brief summaries of key points was something that I relied on when I took the basic science exam. It is a great way to recapitulate key ideas that can be springboards for a deeper dive into areas of study where your feel you need to shore up your knowledge. I have provided such short summaries in this book. They are brief and cryptic statements but have enough information to trigger your own recall of information. Some statements have been repeated for emphasis. They are also presented in a random manner much as how you might encounter the ideas in an exam. You should continue to make notes of your own by jotting down the salient points of the topics that you study. These notes will serve you well.

A word to the wise: Approach the exam in a relaxed and focused way going at about 70 to 90 percent effort level. Don't go at it with a 100 percent as this is not sustainable over the long run. A continually hard-driving pace leads to high stress high levels, and this can have ill health effects. The high tempo may also be counterproductive to sustained attention and enthusiasm. The human body and brain are simply not designed to function well at sustained high stress levels. So 70 to 90 percent is good enough. Draw rough diagrams and sketches and scratch notes that you don't have to show anyone.

The adage of being slow and steady really does apply when it comes to studying for anything. It is a marathon, not the 100-meter dash. Take breaks, look at the trees, birds, and the sky and, try to integrate what you have learned into the larger picture.

I wish you success in this exam and your future career.

T S Gill MD

A LIST OF SHORT SUMMARIES FOLLOWS:

1. Classical Conditioning – In Pavlov's experiment, by pairing the offering of food with the ringing of a bell, a conditioned automatic response occurs in the dog (salivation, secretion of gastric juices) in response to the ringing of the bell even in the absence of the food. Similarly, in chemotherapy, nausea occurs afterward as the patient is exiting in the lobby of the hospital. Next time, the exposure to the lobby causes nausea as a conditioned response even before the chemotherapy has begun.

2. Operant Conditioning – In this type of conditioning, a reward or punishment is used to influence voluntary behaviors. The reward is used to increase behaviors; punishment is used to decrease negative behaviors. There are two types of rewards- negative reinforcement and positive reinforcement.

3. Negative Reinforcement is the removal of an aversive stimulus to reinforce desired behaviors.

4. Positive Reinforcement is the actual giving of a tangible reward or verbal praise to reinforce desired behaviors.

5. Punishment is not ok in therapeutic settings. Positive punishment is aversive stimuli given to decrease unwanted behaviors. An example is the disulfiram reaction in alcoholics when they drink while taking Antabuse. Negative punishment is taking away of a desired object or privilege to decrease unwanted behaviors.

6. The legal and correctional system are based on the expected deterrent effect of punishment on curbing undesirable human behaviors. These punishments can be fines, jail, imprisonment, hard labor and other physical punishments such as hard labor and up to the death penalty. The use of cruel and unusual punishment is specifically forbidden by the Constitution of the United States.

7. Substandard healthcare for prisoners was deemed to be cruel and unusual punishment by a federal court. California prison system and several other states were charged with this violation. Remedial steps were mandated to bring the standard of care in prisons up to the community standards.

8. Extinction- When no reinforcement is given, positive or negative, the behavior tends to decrease and then cease or extinguish.

9. Transference is when patient imposes feelings from his or her past on to the doctor- treats the doctor like the parent that the doctor reminds the patient of.

10. Countertransference- is when the doctor imposes feelings from his or her past on to the patient.

11. One must be aware of such feelings and never act on them. A clue about countertransference can be when a doctor has a strong liking or revulsion towards a patient that they know relatively little about.

12. It is never ok to act out on any romantic feelings that might be aroused towards a patient. This can be grounds for litigation and suspension of license. The rules are very strict in this regard.

13. It is never ok to act out on any strong negative countertransference feelings either by being punitive or abrasive in word or action.

14. If such strong feelings are aroused, it is better to transfer care to another physician.

15. When one is seeing patients of the opposite sex or children, it is always good to have a chaperone in the room. Any allegation of impropriety can end a career, and it is easy for patients to misperceive especially if they have some type of countertransference.

16. Ego Defenses- these are used to protect from a perceived vulnerability.

17. Acting Out- engaging in disruptive or agitated behaviors if feelings are distressful. It is better to exercise, using other coping skills and talk over any conflicts that may exist when one is calm through a prearranged meeting. It is important to explain if you feel disrespected or overlooked or slighted, and the other person will usually be more than happy to make amends. If not, then it is easy to go separate ways in an amicable manner to avoid future strife and grief.

18. Denial- This is a mechanism wherein there is avoidance of acceptance of a painful reality. It is the first stage in coping with loss or grief. It is ok not to puncture this shield that keeps anxiety at bay for the patient. In due time, the person usually will come to accept the reality that seems painful at first.

19. The stages of grief are as follows: DENIAL, ANGER, BARGAINING, DEPRESSION, ACCEPTANCE. The person may cycle back and forth between them a number of times before grief is processed.

20. Elizabeth Kubler-Ross enunciated the stages of grief

21. Displacement- this is kicking the dog syndrome- a person is angry at the boss but is powerless to retaliate so takes it out on his subordinates, spouse, children or pets. This is never a healthy response. Other ways to process frustration are to sublimate it through exercise, laughter, making your faith in a higher power stronger, and other coping strategies.

22. Dissociation – a temporary change in memory, consciousness due to acute or severe chronic stressors. Can lead to fugue state where a person may forget or "lose his identity" and wander off from home or develop multiple identity disorder.

23. Fixation- Undue attachment to childhood behaviors, such as a favorite toy, game, etc. It may help cope and is not totally bad.

24. Idealization – idealizing and thinking only positive thoughts about the other person (putting them on a pedestal) while overlooking their drawbacks. All of us are vulnerable to this if the person is charismatic, but individuals with borderline personality traits or disorder are said to be more likely to idealize.

25. Borderline personality disorder or traits can be a legacy of an abusive or deprived childhood. The person may sometimes lack a strong, coherent sense of their inner self. A strong, charismatic personality can be a beacon of hope and cherished values. The other reaction in borderline personality may be a tendency to categorize individual into all good or all bad categories. Idealization and devaluation are the opposite sides of the same coin.

26. Identification_ modeling oneself after someone more powerful even if one does not totally like them. It may be a good thing if the role model is a healthy one.

27. Intellectualization- This is the psychological act of using rationalization, facts and logic to distance oneself emotionally from a distressing event or situation. The story of the fox and sour grapes is kind of an intellectualization on the part of the Fox.

28. Intellectualization like other psychological defenses is used to shield from the depression of a setback of

some kind. The risk is that the person does not take the initiative to make another attempt at achieving their goal but seals of themselves behind the wall of intellectualization.

29. A part of being a mature adult is the willingness to bear some anxiety and having the courage to take risks in new endeavors knowing that one may not always succeed. Courage is the ability to learn from one's mistakes and try again.

30. Reaction Formation: Behaving in a way opposite of one's feelings. One who is plagued by sexual thoughts and high libido becomes a celibate monk, a person who is corrupt becomes an advocate for ending corruption in the government. One who hates someone expresses feelings of love and shows affection for covering up these feelings.

31. Regression- going back to an earlier stage of development or fixation when under stress. This may include having a movie and video game night and popcorn night and pajama parties of childhood. In children, regression may indicate going back to bedwetting when under stress.

32. Repression- when feelings, memories, and thoughts are outside of awareness and remain in the unconscious parts of the mind due to stressful memories tied to that period. An example is an amnesia for moving away or death of a parent or a period of acute illness. PTSD patients may also repress some memories.

33. Suppression: This is voluntarily deleting negative thoughts from one's mind. This is healthy, and the person is conscious and makes a deliberate choice about what he chooses to bring to his conscious awareness. The ability to suppress is healthy. Not everything has to be talked about or brought into the open if someone does not want to do this.

34. Splitting- Dividing people into all good or bad. People are shades of gray and rarely all good or all bad. In borderline personality disorder, there is a need to idealize, and a tendency exists to categorize people into all good or all bad. People are rarely perfect, and maturity is being able to overlook minor flaws and peccadillos of a person.

35. MATURE DEFENCES ARE LISTED BELOW

    The phrase: Sublime Soup Alters Humor is a way to remember this.

    S- for Sublimation- A negative feeling is mutated into something positive using that drive.- Aggression is turned into excellence in sports or business

    S- Suppression- Voluntarily choosing not to worry about a game until it is time for the game. It can help to improve focus in the now.

    A- For Altruism- negative feelings such as guilt is transformed into charitable acts

    H- Humor- a negative experience is turned into a funny story by seeing the humor in oneself or one's circumstances.

36. Infant Deprivation Effects may lead to a failure to thrive, Lack of well-developed speech, a lack of basic trust, and reactive attachment disorder

37. 40% of deaths in children are those under one year of age

38. Spiral fractures, fractures in multiple stages of healing, beaded rib rosary are signs of physical child abuse. Neglect and verbal abuse often accompany it.

39. Neglect and verbal abuse can also have detrimental effects on the psychological health of the child and the future adult.

40. The biological mother is the most common abuser.

41. Vulnerable Child Syndrome- This is a situation where the concerned parents are overprotective of a child that is sick or has been sick.

42. ADHD onset is before age 12. The main symptoms are limited attention span, hyperactivity, and impulsivity. Treatment is with stimulants methylphenidate, dextroamphetamine, or guanfacine, clonidine, atomoxetine. ADHD from childhood often persists into adulthood in 30 to 50% of the time. Go with 50 percent if it comes as a question in the USMLE test.

43. Autism spectrum disorder- In these disorders, there is an impairment of social relatedness with the outside world. It may be marked by poor eye contact, stereotypical movements, insensitivity to social cues, and impaired communication skills. The severity can vary from mild to severe. It is often accompanied by intellectual handicaps (mental retardation)

44. Rett's disorder- This is an inherited x linked dominant disorder in girls that leads to regression after normal initial development till age 3 or 4. It is later followed by a gradual regression with the loss of speech and the developmental milestones achieved earlier.

45. Conduct Disorder is sometimes a precursor of antisocial personality disorder. In conduct disorder, the normal rules are violated with little remorse. The treatment usually offered is psychotherapy, CBT (cognitive behavioral therapy).

46. Oppositional Defiant Disorder- In this there is usually no major violation of official laws and rules. The children are difficult to handle and may be defiant of the local household rules. The children are usually protesting some social setting where they feel they have been overlooked or ignored and lack trust in adults. Treatment is psychotherapy and CBT

47. Separation Anxiety Disorder- onset around age 7 to 9 or earlier, the child feels harm may come to parent or self, and may be afraid to go to school. Treatment is provided by having the parent going to school for part of the day and gradually increasing the periods of separation. Other interventions may include play therapy and family therapy.

48. Tourette Disorder: Motor and Vocal tics, coprolalia (pt may utter obscenities) that persist for MORE THAN A YEAR. Treatment with antipsychotics fluphenazine or pimozide is helpful. Tetrabenazine, clonidine, guanfacine may also be helpful

49. In Alzheimer's Disease- orientation is lost first to time, then place, then the person.
Memory for long-term memory may be retained to some extent; short-term memory consolidation problems, however, are significant.

50. In delirium, there is a waxing and waning level of alertness, onset is acute and often related to some medical cause such as electrolyte imbalance, hypoxemia, or infection. A diffuse slow wave is often seen on EEG. Treatment should focus on correcting the underlying problem.

51. Dementia is slower in onset and often gradual. *Definitive* Diagnosis of Alzheimer can only be made by a postmortem brain biopsy after death with the recognition of neurofibrillary tangles.

52. Psychosis- is distorted perception of reality caused by hallucinations, delusions.

53. Delusions: These are fixed false beliefs that are impermeable to logic

54. Hallucinations are perceptions in the absence of external stimuli

55. Olfactory hallucinations such as that of burning rubber may occur in epilepsy, brain tumors

56. Gustatory hallucinations may be related to a seizure disorder.

57. Auditory hallucinations are the most common hallucinations in schizophrenia and other psychotic disorders.

58. Hypnagogic hallucinations are those that occur when Going to sleep. May be associated with narcolepsy

59. Schizophrenia marked by positive symptoms of hallucinations, disorganized speech and negative symptoms of avolition (lack of initiative), asocial behaviors, alogia (lack of speech).

60. Negative symptoms of schizophrenia are better targeted by atypical antipsychotics such as risperidone, olanzapine or clozapine.

61. Clozapine is usually reserved for refractory cases because it can cause agranulocytosis.

62. Brief Psychotic Disorder is less than one month

63. Schizophreniform Disorder lasts from 1 month to 6 months

64. Schizophrenia is when psychosis duration is greater than six months

65. Hypnopompic hallucinations occur upon arising from sleep. May be associated with narcolepsy.

66. Schizoaffective Disorder when psychotic and mood disorder symptoms are present together for most of the time.

67. Hypomanic mood is when mood is elevated to a mild degree and does not cause dysfunction

68. Mania is when the mood is significantly elevated and leads to dysfunction due to grandiose ideations and behaviors.

69. Bipolar Disorder is when both depression and manic or hypomanic symptoms alternate. Type I Bipolar has at least one manic episode, Type II Bipolar Disorder never has manic episodes but only hypomanic episodes

70. Cyclothymic Disorder is a milder form bipolar disorder that lasts at least two years.

71. Major Depression is a period sustained a sad mood for at least two weeks and accompanied by at least four symptoms from SIGECAPS to make a total of 5 symptoms. The SIGECAPS symptoms are sleep problems, loss of interest in enjoyable activities, feelings of guilt, decreased energy, concentration is impaired, Appetite may be altered with weight gain or

weight loss, psychomotor activity is decreased, suicidal ideations may be present.

72. Atypical Depression is marked by weight gain, appetite increase and increased sleep.

73. SSRI's are preferred agents to treat depression as they have the least troublesome side effects.

74. MAOI's are effective for Panic Disorder and Atypical Depression but may lead to a hypertensive crisis in the presence of tyramine-containing foods.

75. Postpartum blues are common and occur within 3 to 5 days of childbirth

76. Postpartum depression is more serious and maybe accompanied by psychosis with attendant risk to the newborn and others.

77. Postpartum depression occurs within four months.

78. In grief, some people are profoundly sad, and it may seem as if they are seeing the person at times. It may seem like they hallucinate about the person. This is not pathological.

79. OCD (Obsessive Compulsive Disorder) is marked by intrusive and unwanted thoughts. The person recognizes the irrational nature of the intrusive thoughts and may adopt certain rituals and stereotypical mannerisms to relieve anxiety associated with the intrusive thoughts and

obsessions. Some of these stereotypical behaviors may include washing their hands repeatedly, tapping the table or door in a certain manner, or doing other acts for the same purpose of anxiety relief. Treatment is with high doses of SSRI's and Clomipramine. They all increase serotonin. It can take 6 to 8 weeks of high dose SSRI's to achieve a noticeable benefit for the symptoms.

80. Hypnopompic (hallucinations upon arising) and Hypnagogic (upon falling asleep) hallucinations are usually benign and do not indicate psychosis. They may, however, be associated with other conditions such as narcolepsy.

81. Acute Stress Disorder occurs early after a trauma and can last 30 days after the traumatic event.

82. PTSD occurs after the 30-day duration, marked by intrusive flashbacks, nightmares, startle response. Treatment is with SSRI's.

83. Zero-order elimination – a constant amount of drug is eliminated per unit of time. Elimination Kinetics are a straight line. An example of drugs following this can be remembered by the acronym PEA, P for Phenytoin, E for Ethanol, A for Aspirin. PEA is oval in shape likes like zero by the way

84. First-Order Elimination- The amount of excretion is higher at higher doses, elimination kinetics are a curved line.

85. The way to facilitate excretion for a drug is to make it ionized. This is done by making the urine opposite of the ph of the drug. The ionized drug is not reabsorbed and is excreted.

86. Weakly acidic drugs like aspirin, methotrexate, phenobarbital are excreted more when the urine is made alkaline by giving the patient bicarbonate

87. Drugs that are weak bases such as Tricyclic Antidepressants, amphetamines are excreted more if the urine is made acidic by giving ammonium chloride.

88. Phase 1 reactions are oxidation, reduction, hydrolysis

89. Phase II reactions are conjugation reactions that make the drugs polar and ionized and are more readily excreted.

90. Efficacy is different from potency. Efficacy is a true level of greater benefit for alleviating symptoms of an illness.

91. Potency just means less of a drug is needed to achieve a certain physiologic or pharmacodynamics effect. The amount of effect is, however, the same and potency does not necessarily denote greater efficacy or therapeutic effect.

92. Therapeutic Index is Dose that is toxic in 50 percent of individuals divided by dose that is effective in 50 % of individuals. It is TD50/ED 50

93. Cholinesterase Inhibitor found in insecticides. Toxicity can cause a cholinergic syndrome (Diarrhea, Urination, Miosis (constriction of pupils), Lacrimation, and Salivation) and can be lethal. The antidote is anticholinergic Atropine (competitive inhibitor), and Pralidoxime. Pralidoxime can help regenerate the cholinesterase.

94. Muscarinic Antagonists are also called Anticholinergics

95. Some of these drugs include atropine, benztropine (used for parkinsonian side effects with antipsychotic medications), glycopyrrolate (given to preoperative bronchial, oral secretions), ipratropium (used in COPD, asthma), dicyclomine (antispasmodics for GI), oxybutynin, solifenacin, tolterodine for urinary bladder frequency. One should always search and rule out any underlying medical causes such as a urinary tract infection before offering merely symptomatic treatment with these agents.

96. Many agents can have anticholinergic effects, and they can add up and cause anticholinergic toxicity especially in the elderly.

97. If an elderly person is confused, with fast heart rate, dry mucous membranes, check medication regimen for possible anticholinergic medications or medications with anticholinergic side effects. Datura poisoning also causes an anticholinergic delirium.

The way to remember the effects of **anticholinergic** medications toxicity is using the mnemonic *Hot as a hare, blind as a bat, dry as a bone, red as a beet, mad as a hatter.*

98. **Hot as a hare**: increased body temperature

99. **Blind as a bat**: mydriasis (dilated pupils)

100. **Dry as a bone**: dry mouth, dry eyes, decreased sweat

101. **Red as a beet**: flushed face

102. **Mad as a hatter**: delirium

103. Histamine poisoning (also called scombroid poisoning) is related to eating spoiled dark meat fish (tuna, mahi-mahi, bonito, mackerel). The bacterial enzyme histidine decarboxylase converts the histidine in fish to histamine. Symptoms include flushing, erythema, bronchospasm, may resemble an anaphylactic reaction. Treatment is with antihistamines, albuterol and epinephrine if needed. May be confused with a true allergy to fish.

104. Ciguatoxin is found in some reef fish such as barracuda, snapper, and moray eel. The toxin causes depolarization by opening Na channel. Treatment is supportive. May resemble cholinergic poisoning.

105. Tetrodotoxin is found in puffer fish and is very deadly, prevents depolarization. Treatment is supportive.

TOXINS AND ANTIDOTES

106. Acetaminophen- N-acetylcysteine

107. Acetylcholinesterase inhibitors (organophosphates)- Atropine +Pralidoxime

108. Amphetamines- Give ammonium chloride to increase excretion, manage hypertension, anxiety, agitation as indicated with other meds

109. Anticholinergic toxicity- physostigmine, control hyperthermia

110. Arsenic- Dimercaprol, succimer

111. Benzodiazepines- antidote is flumazenil. The dose may have to be repeated because of short half-life. Supportive care

112. Beta blockers- saline, atropine, glucagon. Glucagon works by a unique mechanism and can help when beta blocker overdose has caused braycardia (slowed heart rate).

113. Carbon Monoxide- 100 percent oxygen, hyperbaric oxygen.

114. Copper- as in Wilson's disease- pencilliamine, trientine

115. Cyanide- Nitrite, thiosulfate, hydroxycobalamin

116. Digitoxin- Antidigitalis Fab fragments

117. Gold- Penicillamine, Dimercaprol (BAL), Succimer

118. Heparin- Protamine Sulfate

119. Iron- Desferrioxamine, defrasinox, deferiprone

120. Lead- EDTA, Dimercaprol, Pencillamine, Succimer

121. Mercury- Dimercaprol, succimer

122. Methanol, Ethylene chloride (antifreeze) – Fomepizole, Ethanol, Dialysis

123. Methemoglobinemia- Methylene blue, Vitamin C

124. Opioids- Naloxone IM, or intranasal- may need to be repeated due to short half-life, supportive care

125. Salicylates- Sodium bicarbonate to increase excretion

126. TCA- Sodium bicarbonate to increase excretion

127. Coumadin- Vit K for delayed benefit, fresh frozen plasma for more immediate benefit.

128. Cardiovascular Drug Reactions are below

129. Coronary Vasospasm- sumatriptan (used for migraines), ergot alkaloids (used for migraines), cocaine (abused drug)

130. Ergot alkaloids have also been associated with gangrene in limbs, fingers due to severe vasospasm.

131. Cutaneous Flushing – remembered with acronym VANCE: V for vancomycin (slow infusion may prevent this), Adenosine (short acting, used to terminate cardiac arrhythmias- very effective), and Niacin (can be prevented by aspirin), Ca Channel blockers, and Echinocandins (antifungal drugs e.g., Micafungin)

132. Dilated Cardiomyopathy-

Anthracyclines

(Chemotherapeutic agents uses for breast cancer such as Doxorubicin, daunorubicin)- prevent with dexrazoxane

133. Torsade's de Pointes- undulating EKG line, the arrhythmia is related to prolonged conduction time within the heart. It can degenerate into a fatal ventricular fibrillation. Agents that can cause this are remembered with following simple acronym. ABCDE

A for Antiarrhythmics Type Ia and Type III

B for Antibiotics- macrolide such as erythromycin, azithromycin- they displace other agents and can raise levels to cause toxic side effects

C for Antipsy©hotics such as haloperidol and others at high doses, also lithium

D- Antidepressants such as TCA (Tricyclic Antidepressants) and citalopram at higher doses

E- Antiemetic's such as ondansetron

134. Adrenocortical Insufficiency- Due to withdrawal from external glucocorticoids- this is the most common cause

135. Hot Flashes- Methotrexate (chemotherapy), clomiphene (fertility drug used to induce ovulation- this is, by the way, the most common cause of multiple pregnancies like twin, triplets or more)

136.　　Hyperglycemia – remembered with acronym: TAKING PILLS NECESSITATES HAVING BLOOD CHECKED SURELY

T for Tacrolimus (An immunosuppressant used to prevent rejection of donated organs)

P- Protease Inhibitors (e.g.,. Zidovudine used to treat HIV infection)

N- Niacin

H- HCTZ (hydrochlorothiazide diuretic for hypertension)

C – Corticosteroids

S- Second-generation antipsychotics can cause hyperglycemia due to inducing insulin resistance. They also can cause metabolic syndrome (weight gain, increased cholesterol, insulin resistance)

137. Hypothyroidism can be caused by Lithium, Amiodarone, Sulfonamides

138.　　Acute cholestatic hepatitis, jaundice – can be related to erythromycin

139. Focal to Massive Hepatic Necrosis- can occur with Halothane, Death Cap Mushroom poisoning (amanita phalloides), Valproic acid, acetaminophen

140.　　Diarrhea can be a side effect of SSRI (sertraline-Zoloft), orlistat (prevents fat absorption-used for weight control), metformin (used for diabetes, starting drug, does not cause hypoglycemia, can cause lactic acidosis), misoprostol (used to protect from peptic ulcer formation when NSAIDs are used, also used along with mifepristone to induce abortion), quinidine (antiarrhythmic), ezetimibe (given to lower cholesterol by preventing cholesterol absorption from gi tract)

141. Hepatitis- Rifampin, Isoniazid, Pyrazinamide- all three are to treat TB, Statins (to treat high cholesterol), fibrates- (used for hyperlipidemia)

142. Pancreatitis causing drugs can be remembered by the sentence – DRUGS CAUSING A VIOLENT ABDOMINAL DISTRESS

D - Didanosine (used to treat HIV infection)

C - Corticosteroids

A -Alcohol

V - Valproic Acid (used to treat seizure disorder, bipolar disorder)

A – Azathioprine- (It is used as an immunosuppressant used to treat Rheumatoid arthritis and rejection of kidney or other donated organs)

D- Diuretics (Furosemide, HCTZ)

143.Pill Induced Esophagitis- Tetracycline, Bisphosphonates (used to treat osteoporosis, is a very big risk, person told not to recline for at least half an hour afterward) , Potassium Chloride (This should always be given with a large glass of water to avoid GI distress in the esophagus and stomach)

144. Pseudomembranous Enterocolitis: Clindamycin, Ampicillin, Cephalosporins more commonly associated with this.

They predispose to overgrowth of Clostridium difficile. Use of cultured yogurt may provide some protection.

145.Agranulocytosis: The following agents may cause it: Clozapine (Second Generation Antipsychotic used for refractory psychosis), Carbamazepine (used for seizure disorder, bipolar disorder), Propylthiouracil (used to treat Hyperthyroidism – Grave's Disease- it inhibits conversion of thyroxine to triiodothyronine T3 in peripheral tissues- used along with surgery , Methimazole (also used for treating hyperthyroidism), Colchicine (used to treat acute gout), Ganciclovir (antiviral acyclic nucleoside used to treat herpes, CMV, and CMV- it inhibits the replication of the viruses)

146.   Aplastic Anemia: Caused by Carbamazepine, Methimazole, NSAIDS, Benzene, Chloramphenicol, Propylthiouracil

147. Direct Coombs Positive hemolytic anemia- caused by methyldopa, penicillin

(these drugs cause development of antibodies to the Rh antigen or the antibiotic/cell membrane complex and this leads to hemolysis.

148.   Gray Baby Syndrome: Chloramphenicol is contraindicated in infancy. The liver in infancy lacks the necessary enzymes required to metabolize chloramphenicol. The accumulation of chloramphenicol leads to adverse effects such as hypotension and an ashen appearance marked by cyanosis in lips, nail beds and skin from hypoxemia.

149.   Hemolysis in G6PD deficiency: Remembered by the acronym: Hemolysis IS D PAIN

I-   Isoniazid- used to treat TB, needs B6 supplementation

S- Sulfonamide- antibiotic

D- Dapsone- used to treat leprosy, prevention of toxoplasmosis in immune compromised

P- Primaquine- Primaquine phosphate is prescribed to eradicate infection by plasmodium vivax.

A- Aspirin

I-   Ibuprofen

N- Nitrofurantoin (used to treat UTI)

150.   Glucose-6-phosphate dehydrogenase deficiency is a genetic disorder that occurs most often in males. This condition mainly affects red blood cells, which carry oxygen from the lungs to tissues throughout the body. In affected individuals, a defect in an enzyme called glucose-6-phosphate dehydrogenase causes red blood cells to break down prematurely. This destruction of red blood cells is called hemolysis. In people with glucose-6-dehydrogenase deficiency, hemolytic anemia is most often triggered by bacterial or viral infections or by

certain drugs (such as some antibiotics and medications used to treat malaria). Hemolytic anemia can also occur after eating fava beans or inhaling pollen from fava plants (a reaction called favism).

151. Megaloblastic Anemia- Phenytoin, Methotrexate, Sulfa drugs

152. Thrombocytopenia- Heparin

153. Thrombotic Complications- Oral Contraceptive, Hormone replacement therapy (both androgens and estrogens)

154. Fat Redistribution- Protease inhibitors, Glucocorticoids

155. Gingival Hyperplasia- Phenytoin, Ca Channel blockers, cyclosporine (used as an immunosuppressive for treatment of Rheumatoid Arthritis, Psoriasis, and to prevent organ rejection)

156. Hyperuricemia – caused by some drugs - remembered by the phrase PAINFUL TOPHI AND FEET NEED CARE

P- Pyrazinamide (for TB)

T- Thiazide

F- Furosemide

N-Niacin

C – Cyclosporine

157. Myopathy: Fibrates, Niacin, Colchicine, Hydroxychloroquine, Interferon alpha, penicillamine

158.   Penicillamine "is used as a chelating agent in the following conditions.

- In Wilson's disease - a rare genetic disorder of copper metabolism, penicillamine treatment relies on its binding to accumulated copper and elimination through urine.[1]
- In cystinuria, penicillamine is helpful. This is a hereditary disorder featuring formation of cysteine stones. Penicillamine binds with cysteine to form a disulfide that is more water soluble and excreted without precipitation as stones.
- Penicillamine has been used also to treat scleroderma as well.
- Penicillamine has been used in the past for arsenic poisoning, but Dimercaprol is now the preferred therapy for Arsenic toxicity.

159.   Osteoporosis – can be caused by corticosteroids, heparin

160.   Photosensitivity- remembered by phrase SAT

For PHOTO

S- Sulfonamides

A-   Amiodarone – antiarrhythmic

T – Tetracycline

5- FU is a chemotherapy agent

161. Rash- (Steven Johnson Syndrome)- Antiepileptic drugs (especially lamotrigine), allopurinol, sulfa drugs, penicillin

162. SLE like syndrome- Sulfa drugs, Hydralazine, Isoniazid, Procainamide (antiarrhythmic), Phenytoin, Etanercept - REMEMBERED BY PHRASE IS 'SHIPPE."

163. Systemic Lupus Erythematosus is an autoimmune disease which can affect many different organ systems. The course of the disease can be unpredictable and can have a waxing and waning course.

164. (Enbrel) is a medication that is helpful for treating autoimmune disease. It acts by being an inhibitor of the tumor necrosis factor. It is helpful with rheumatoid arthritis, psoriatic arthritis, and ankylosing spondylitis.

165. Teeth Discoloration can occur if tetracyclines are prescribed to children.

166. Tendonitis, tendon rupture, and cartilage damage- Fluoroquinolones

167. Cinchonism: is caused by an overdose of quinidine. It is marked by ringing in ears (tinnitus), blurred vision, and prolongation of myocardial conduction time as manifested by increased duration of QTc as measured on the EKG. It is derived from its natural source the cinchona bark.

Tardive Dyskinesia- Antipsychotics, metoclopramide

168. Parkinsonism-like syndrome – Antipsychotics, reserpine, metoclopramide – Antipsychotics and metoclopramide cause dopamine receptor blockade causes it, also caused by metoclopramide – same mechanism, reserpine – depletes catecholamines like dopamine. Reserpine can also lead to severe depression due to the same reasons and is contraindicated in those with a history of depression, is not used much anymore

169. Diabetes Insipidus- may be induced by Lithium and demeclocycline

170. Lithium is a salt that is used to treat bipolar disorder; demeclocycline is a tetracycline antibiotic that is now used infrequently to treat bacterial infections. They can both cause diabetes insipidus.

171. Demeclocycline has an anti-ADH effect and is used potentially to treat SIADH.

172. SIADH (Syndrome of Inappropriate (excessive effect) antidiuretic hormone) leads to water retention. This leads to dilution of electrolytes (hyponatremia) and increased blood volume.

173. SIADH can present as weakness, confusion, and delirium.

174. Correction of hyponatremia must be gradual. Too rapid a correction can lead to neurological complications through a condition called central pontine myelinolysis (CMP).

175. Fanconi Syndrome- Tenofovir – antiretroviral for HIV infection, ifosamide (chemotherapeutic agent to treat cancer)

176. Fanconi Syndrome- This is a syndrome affecting the proximal tubule in which there is leakage of glucose, amino acids, uric acid, bicarbonate, and phosphate. It is associated with heredity and sometimes with exposure to certain drugs and heavy metals.

177. Interstitial Cystitis- Methicillin, NSAIDS, Furosemide

178. SIADH- SSRI, cyclophosphamide, Carbamazepine

179. A dry cough can be caused by- Ace Inhibitors like captopril, Lisinopril used to treat hyertnsion

180. Pulmonary Fibrosis- Methotrexate, Nitrofurantoin, Carmustine, Bleomycin, Busulfan, Amiodarone to remember phrase MY NOSE CAN NOT BREATHE BAD AIR

181. Carmustine is a medication used for chemotherapy and for immunosuppression sometimes to decrease risk for donated organ rejection.

182. Positive predictive value of test increases when the prevalence of a disease is high, the negative predictive value increases when the prevalence is low.

183. The sensitivity and specificity are not affected by prevalence.

184. Z score means the number of standard deviations from the mean.

185. Specificity is the likelihood of a test being negative when there is no disease

186. Case-control studies look backward to see "what happened to cause disease."

187. Cohort studies look forward to see who will develop disease when different persons are exposed to different risk factors.

188. An accurate test is a test that yields results close to reality. A "precise test" just reproduces the results without much deviation upon repeat testing. It may or may not be close to reality. The best test is both accurate and precise.

189. If a test with high specificity is positive, it helps to RULE IN disease (SPIN- specificity rules in disease)

190. Adoption studies help to determine the effect of genetic and environmental factors by studying siblings or twins in adoptive and home settings.

191. Phases of study PHASE I- trial in a small number of healthy people, PHASE II- a study in a small number of people with the target disease, PHASE III- Larger number of people randomly assigned to either test drug or placebo PHASE IV- performance after the test drug has entered the market. Rare side effects may only come to light in the last phase of PHASE IV when a large number of people have been exposed.

192. Trick Question- Calculating percentile with standard deviations. 2 standard deviation includes the middle 95%. The bottom of the 2 SD is at 2.5 percentile, and the top of the two standard deviations is 97.5 percentile.

193. When asked to calculate percentile in a person who is two standard deviations above the mean- you take the 95 percent of the middle area of the 2 SD and add the lower 2.5 percent to get a percentile of 97.5 %

194.   Communities are separate, and this data about communities is called nominal or categorical.

195.   Confounding variables are those make it difficult to determine the cause.

196.   Selection bias is when a representative population is not chosen

197. Late look bias is when the sickest individuals are excluded because they die off early in a study and are excluded.

198. Pygmalion effect is when the experimenter's expectations are inadvertently communicated to the subject and the subject who then tries to report the desired effect.(This is overcome by preferably double blinding the study- neither the experimenter or the subject knows who is getting the real drug)

199. Injuries occur more often in men compared to women. Injuries are the top 5 causes of death in men.

200. The crude mortality rate is all deaths per a population for a time period- usually per year.

201. A metaanalysis is when results from different studies are combined and analyzed

202. Positive predictive value is true positive divided by all positives

203. Negative predictive values is true negatives divided by all negatives

204. A case study is the write-up of physical findings, other info, history and course of an illness that is rare. It can be very useful

205. Type I error- false alarm error- a researcher reports a finding as significant when it is not but just a chance variation

206.   Power is the ability to detect a true difference when a difference exists. The power of a study should be set at a minimum of 80%.

207.   The power of a test is 100 minus whatever beta is. If the beta is 20 percent, Power is 100 minus 20 or 80 percent.

208.   The power of a test is increased if the effect size is large or the sample size is large.

209.   HIPPA laws protect coverage for pregnancy, changing jobs, moving or divorce. It also provides for confidentiality of medical records and the obligation to protect the confidentiality.

210. If patients select themselves for a group, this is selection bias

211. Case-control studies look at a group of people with a disease and then compare them with people without a disease.

212. Relative risk is determined by cohort studies, not case-control studies. This is because there is a better ideas of the risk factors going forward in a cohort studies.

213. To qualify for hospice care, the criterion is a medically anticipated death within six months.

214. Prevalence is the number of people with the disease in a given population.

215. The p-value is a measure of making a type I error (raising a false alarm).

216. If the p value is 0.05, it means there is only a 5 percent chance of making a type I error- at this level, the finding is considered clinically significant.

217. The most important characteristic of a screening test is high sensitivity.

218. The most important characteristic of a confirmatory test is high specificity.

219. Selection bias is overcome by randomization

220. The "Pygmalion Effect," is when people start to act or respond in a way that they think they are expected to respond.— a person expected by his or her superiors to succeed will succeed, but if he is expected in his mind to fail, the subject will find a way to fail.

221. Most of the time, these expectations from the experimenter are not openly expressed but may be communicated passively through body language or slips of the tongue or word choice.

222. The Hawthorne effect occurs when a researcher is observing the person in a study In this effect, the subject under study tends to increase the behavior he or she thinks is desirable by the

researcher. This tends to confound the objectivity of the results.

223.   Hawthorne effect is also seen in work settings. When workers feel like they are being observed, he or she tends to increase behavior they think is desirable.

224.   Both the Pygmalion and Hawthorne effect are overcome by double blinding (neither the experimenter nor the subject knows which drug the person is getting).

225.   Independent variables are those that the experimenter controls such as the intake of salt by a subject and dependent variable is the outcome that is measured such as blood pressure.

226.   A mammogram as screening is an example of secondary prevention. All screening is secondary prevention- to detect disease early

227.   Exercise, avoidance of smoking, a vegetarian diet is an example of primary prevention.

228.   Tertiary prevention is treatment at hospital and rehab to reduce disability.

229.   Type II error rate is =false negatives (failure to raise alarm, failure to recognize positive) divided by all true positives

230.	The power of an experiment is the ability to detect a significant effect when one exists. It is improved if the effect size is large or the sample number is large.

231. The case-specific mortality in above is number of deaths among those that have the disease which is 500. So case-specific mortality is 50/500 (choice C)

232.	One way to remember is that cause is a longer word than case, so cause-specific mortality is the no. of deaths over the larger number 100,000. Case specific goes with the shorter number of 500, so case-specific mortality is 50/100

233.	Sensitivity is the ability of the test to detect a disease or the likelihood of a test being positive when the disease is present.

234.	BMI is calculated by height in meters divided by wt in KG squared M (Meters) / Kg*Kg

235.	Odds Ratio is calculated as follows:

All true multiplied with each other divided by All False multiplied with each other

Or

True Positive X False Negative /divided/ by False Positive X True Negative

236. **Type I** error is a **false alarm error**- someone says findings are significant when they are not. Null hypothesis is falsely rejected in reality the null is true, there is no significant difference.

237. **Type II** error is when **there is no alarm when there should be** (findings are significant)

238. ALL POSITIVE are Those that the tests detected (positive) + All those missed by the test (False negatives)

239. Positive predictive value is those who test positive divided by ALL POSITIVE as described in above (those who test positive + those that are positive but missed - false negative)

240. The divorce rate in the United States is 50%

241. Medicaid is insurance for the poor. It has both federal and state run components. It is run by the state for poor people but has some funding from the federal level.

242. Reliability of a test is when the test yields the same result in different settings. It is a measure of reproducibility. Reproducibility is different from validity. Something can be reproducible but may not be valid.

243. Two measures such as wt and blood pressure when they increase together are said to have a positive correlation.

244. When they move in opposite direction, it is a negative correlation; these are measured by the correlation coefficient. The perfect correlation is a -1 or +1

245. 95% confidence is mean it lies within two standard errors of the mean

246. Standard Error is Standard Deviation divided by the square root of the total number of patients.

247. 95 % confidence interval is mean +- 2 standard errors

248. The t-test is used to compare the means of two groups

249. ANOVA is used to test and compare means of more than two groups

250. Chi-square is used to compare a nominal variable in two groups

251. When one variable increases and the other does not, there is zero correlation.

252. When both increase with each other, there is a positive correlation. The closer the value is to 1, the greater is the correlation

253. When one increases and the other decreases, it is a negative correlation. The closer the correlation value is to negative 1, the greater is the correlation.

254. Correlation does not necessarily mean cause and effect. Something else could be causing both to increase in response to a third factor.

255. Prevalence is the number of people with the disease (True Positives+ False Negatives) divided by the total number of individuals in the population studied.

256. A cohort study selects a group of individuals and studies them for the emergence of a disease, or whatever else is being studied.

257. Hepatitis B and AIDS are reportable. HIV infection is not reportable

258. AIDS is a condition due to HIV infection when the T cell count falls below 200.

259. Reporting laws may vary by state

260. When results of a test are in a tight cluster, the result is said to be precise

261. If vegetable consumption goes up and cancer rates go down, it is said to be a negative correlation (one is going up, the other is going down)

262. Selection bias is eliminated by randomization of the assignment of subjects for different treatment.

263. Primary prevention is the prevention of disease. Secondary prevention is the early detection and treatment of the disease. Tertiary treatment is the treatment at advanced centers and limitation of the disability.

264. The greatest reward for healthcare efforts is at primary prevention.

265. Type II error is also called beta error – <u>alarm is not raised when it </u>should be when the result findings are significant. Type II error just lets it be-ta

266. Type I error is when there is a false alarm of significance when it is really not

267. The confidence of a test is also called the power of the test- synonymous

268. Sensitivity is the ability of the test to detect a disease when it is present.

269. The definition of obese is a body mass index greater than 30.

270. Positive Predictive value of a test is the ratio of true positives divided by all positive tests. So if in a population of 75 patients that test positive and only 60 have the illness, the positive predictive value will be 60/75

271. The t-test is used to compare means of data between two groups such as cholesterol values between men and women.

272.   Teenage marriage, mixed religions, and low socioeconomic status are risk factors for divorce.

273.   The best way to avoid Type I errors (false alarm errors) is to increase the specificity of the test.

274.   A z-score is the measure of the distance in terms of standard deviation from the mean.

275.   The primary source of calories during fasting for the first five days is fat

276.   In prolonged starvation, the primary source of energy is ketone bodies. For the brain, ketones become an important source of fuel after two days

277.   The risk for squamous cell carcinoma of the head and neck is increased 35 fold when alcohol and tobacco are used by a person. They act synergistically as a carcinogen and the risk of exposure together is synergistic and higher than just additive risk.

278.   Users of smokeless chewing tobacco have four times the risk of oral cancer.

279.   SSSS is Staphylococcal Scalded Skin Syndrome is caused by an exfoliative exotoxin that causes a cleavage plan in the epidermis layer of the epidermis. Infection is in otitis media is the site of the primary

infection. This exfoliative exotoxin is produced by some Staphylococcus aureus strains. The intensity of this reaction can vary and may raise suspicions of child abuse due to exposure to hot liquids that have scaled the skin.

280.   Treatment is with fluid, electrolyte replacement, and preventing infection similar to burn injury management.

281. Toxic Epidermal Necrolysis (TEN) is a severe type of immune reaction to dermoepidermal layers of skin in response various medications such as phenytoin, sulfonamides, tetracyclines, and barbiturates. It is not a reaction to an infection. There can be dermal detachment on more than 30 percent of the body surface, the equivalent of second-degree burn.

282.   When this immune reaction affects less than 10 percent of the area, it is called Steven Johnson syndrome. In Steven Johnson syndrome, respiratory and alimentary epithelial sloughing may also occur leading to respiratory failure and malabsorption.

283.   May need treatment in a specialized burn unit to manage and avoid complications.

284. Neurons and heart cells are permanent cells. Are not replaced if lost. That is why heart attacks and strokes lead to enduring decline in function.

285. Emboli from the carotid often go to the distribution of the middle cerebral artery.

286. Subacute Thyroiditis (de Quervain's syndrome) is thought to be of viral origin mediated autoimmune reaction.

287. SLE is a type III reaction with DNA antibody and antibodies to Sm (Smith) antigen, also malar rash, arthralgia, hilar adenopathy, more in AA women

288. In tension pneumothorax, air can enter the pleural space but cannot exit

289. Marked elevation of AFP occurs in hepatocellular carcinoma and teratocarcinoma.

290. The most effective treatment for thrombotic thrombocytopenic purpura (TTP) is plasmapheresis. Rituximab, a monoclonal antibody against the CD 20 protein on B lymphocytes is also used.

291. Platelet infusions in TTP are contraindicated.

292. Thyroid lymphoma treated with chemotherapy and radiation

293. Staphylococcal scalded skin syndrome is associated with staphylococcus infection of otitis media

294.   Plasmapheresis is a procedure used to replace the plasma to remove antibodies that may be involved in an autoimmune disease.

295.   T-Cells and Macrophages are involved in a positive TB test which is a Type IV reaction.

296.   Turner syndrome has a 45XO karyotype with a missing X chromosome. The phenotype (external appearance) characteristics are a webbed neck, short stature, amenorrhea, higher risk for coarctation of the aorta.

297.   A Barr body is an inactive X chromosome. In the case of Turner Syndrome, the Barr body is absent because there is only one X chromosome.

        .

298.   Prostacyclin PG1-1 is a prostaglandin that causes vasodilation and is a platelet antiaggregant. It is produced in the endothelial cells.

299.   It is a product of the cyclooxygenase pathway of arachidonic acid; aspirin inhibits this pathway.

300.   Thromboxane A2 OR (TX A2) is produced by the platelets and is a vasoconstrictor and a platelet aggregant.

301.   Ventricular tachycardia is three beats or more at a rate greater than 100 beats per minute

302.　Disorder of the semicircular canals causes vertigo

303.　Bile produced by the liver helps in the absorption of Vit D. the 25 hydroxylation occurs in the liver, the 1 hydroxylation in the kidney to produce the active form of Vit D (1, 25 dihydroxycholecalciferol).

304.　New onset of glucose intolerance in a patient on TPN (total parenteral nutrition) can be due to chromium deficiency. Other deficiencies can occur, zinc deficiency and lead to an eczematous rash, copper, iron deficiency associated with microcytic anemia.

305.　The von Willebrand factor is required for the platelets to adhere to the subendothelium of the injured vessel wall. A deficiency of the Von Willebrand factor leads to prolonged bleeding times.

306.　Partial albinism and bleeding disorder are associated with dense granule disease

307.　The predominant cell in the first 24 hours of a wound is the PMN's (Polymorphonuclear leukocyte- white blood cell)

308.　The peak time for fibroblasts is six days after the injury

309.　The primary function of macrophages in wound healing is activation of cell proliferation. They also keep the wound clean (wound debridement) and fight infection via oxygen radical and nitric oxide synthesis.

310. The first cells to move into the wound are PMN's.

311. Type I and Type III collagen are important in wound healing.

312. TGF- beta is an important cytokine mediator of wound healing.

313. Chronic use of glucocorticoids leads to decreased collagen synthesis and decreased wound strength.

314. Vitamin A should be given to those receiving corticosteroids to promote wound healing.

315. Zollinger-Ellison Syndrome is associated with increased gastric acid production, hypercalcemia, and malignancy.

316. Carbamazepine can cause aplastic anemia.

433. In Aplastic Anemia, the bone marrow is hypocellular without any abnormal cells.

434. Other causes of aplastic anemia are: Epstein Barr Virus

Hep C, Parvovirus B 19, benzene, insecticides, and chemotherapy drugs or idiopathic (without identified cause)

317. Alcohol can suppress bone marrow and affect all cell lines. It should not be at the top of the differential when carbamazepine is also an alternative choice.

318. Pernicious Anemia is due to intrinsic factor absence related b12 deficiency; It only affects the erythrocytes and not the other cell lines.

319. The TB test is a type IV hypersensitivity test and is mediated by T cells and macrophages.

320. In the above type IV reaction, the T cells are converted to TH1 cells that activates interferon gamma which is the central mediator of the delayed hypersensitivity.

437 T Helper cells type 1 associated with cell-mediated immunity in response to intracellular bacteria and viruses. Produce interferon gamma, interleukin2 and tumor necrosis factor which activates macrophages

438. T Helper cells type 2 are associated with other interleukins IL4, 5, 10 and 13 which stimulate antibody production, eosinophil activation, and other effects on macrophages. T helper 2 cell response is more predominant in gastrointestinal nematode infestation.

439. Long standing hypertension leads to hypertrophy of the left ventricle (the muscle has to pump against increased blood pressure). In this, the size of individual cells is increased.

440. Very high triglyceride levels are a risk factor for acute pancreatitis.

441. After surgery for parathyroid glands, there may be what is called bone hunger. The bones which have been drained of calcium due to the high levels of parathyroid hormone attract the calcium for the next 2 to 3 days to make up some of the deficit. The process eventually settles after 3 to 4 days but for the initial few days, there may be mild hypocalcemia due to this "bone hunger."

442. Hypomagnesaemia resembles hypocalcemia. And both result in increased deep tendon reflexes. Hypokalemia on the other hand causes decreased tendon reflexes

443. Hypocalcaemia can also cause carpopedal spasm and tetany.

444. Acute hypophosphatemia is associated with that refeeding syndrome.

445. Refeeding Syndrome consists of metabolic disturbance that can occur if severely malnourished individuals are reintroduced to a full regular diet without a gradual increase in nutritional intake.

446. In cases where hypokalemia is associated with hypomagnesemia- it is important to replace the magnesium as well in order to get an adequate correction of the hypokalemia state.

447. Alkalosis tends to cause a decrease in potassium (due to excretion by the kidneys of potassium for retention of H ions to correct the alkalosis)

448. Normovolemic hyponatremia is related to SIADH

449. Hypervolemic Hyponatremia associated with polydipsia (water toxicity)

450. Hypothermia can initiate the neuroendocrine response of shock- adrenal medulla releases catecholamines

451. In hypovolemic shock, there is a movement of interstitial fluid into intracellular fluid. Also, the cell membranes become more permeable to sodium.

452. The initiating event in shock is cellular energy deficit.

453. Hypoxia at the cellular level decreases ATP production. This changes intracellular calcium signaling.

454. In bacterial pneumonia, the neutrophils would be the most prominent white blood cells coming to fight off the infection.

455. Streptococcus pneumoniae is the most common cause of lobar pneumonia.

456. Atypical lobular hyperplasia increases the risk for breast cancer.

457. The absence of breasts is associated with the Poland syndrome.

458. Klippel-Trenaunay syndrome is associated with capillary venous and lymphatic malformations.

459. The most common cause of hepatic abscess in the United States is biliary tract procedures.

460. The presence of a solitary star shaped pulmonary nodule with linear strands going outward for 4 to 5 mm is called Corona radiata (radiating star shaped nodule). This is a classic sign of lung cancer.

461. About 25% of all cancers in men and 53% of the lung cancers in women are not related to smoking. They are often adenocarcinomas.

462. Lung cancer in a person who has never smoked is most likely to be an adenocarcinoma. They can be associated with paraneoplastic syndromes.

463. In Marfan syndrome, the protein Fibrillin is defective.

464. A Marjolin ulcer arises in an area exposed to thermal injury.

465. Marjolin's Ulcer refers to a squamous cell carcinoma that develops in areas of chronic irritation or trauma and ulcerates. Such areas can be chronic wounds, burn injuries, or chronic irritation from any cause.

466. A biopsy is recommended first in such a type of ulcer is suspected.

---

467. A germ cell tumor is more likely to be found in the anterior mediastinum.

468. Schwannomas are more likely to be found in the paravertebral areas.

469. Schwannomas and neurofibrosarcomas are tumors of the nerve sheaths that coat the nerve fibers. Schwannomas tend to be benign; neurofibrosarcomas tend to be malignant.

470. A Schwannoma of the vestibulocochlear nerve is called an acoustic neuroma. It causes tinnitus and hearing loss on that side.

471. Ret proto-oncogene on Chromosome 10 is associated with familial medullary thyroid cancer. Also associated with MEN IIa and MEN II b

472. The syndrome of multiple endocrine neoplasias is comprised of different syndromes.

473. Below are some useful hints to remember the different syndromes.

   MEN I **(3 Ps)** - Pituitary, Parathyroid, Pancreatic

   MEN IIa **(1 M, 2 P)** - Medullary Thyroid Ca, Phaeochromocytoma, Parathyroid tumor

   MEN IIb **(2Ms, 1P)** - Medullary Thyroid Ca, Marfanoid Habitus /mucosal neuroma, Pheochromocytoma

474. Medullary thyroid cancer is associated with hyperparathyroidism.

475. Calcitonin levels are useful for diagnosing medullary thyroid cancer. Calcitonin levels are elevated in the presence of the medullary thyroid cancer.

476. The lack of intrinsic factor leads to malabsorption of vitamin B12

   This leads to low vitamin B12 levels which can lead to anemia (called Pernicious Anemia), neuropathy.

   The RBC's are enlarged (macrocytosis). The methylmalonic acid level is elevated if macrocytosis is due to B12 deficiency (it is a coenzyme with B12 and tries to compensate). Folate deficiency also causes macrocytosis but in this case, the methylmalonic acid level will be normal and is NOT elevated.

   The neuropathy due to B12 deficiency may cause postural hypotension and a positive Romberg sign.

477. Romberg's test or sign: A patient with neuropathy has impaired proprioception due to impairment of the conduction from the peripheral nerves. Normally balance is maintained by compensation with vision and vestibular function. When vision is taken away by asking the patient to close their eyes, the person may begin to sway.

478. Romberg Test can be positive in the following illnesses.

B12 neuropathy, Tabes Dorsalis due to neurosyphilis (where it was first noticed), Friedreich's Ataxia, demyelinating diseases, and Meniere's disease.

479. Tactile cells or Merkel cells or Markel-Ranvier cells are oval in shape and found in the skin. They provide somatosensory feedback of light touch through afferent nerves. A malignant tumor of these cells can occur and is called a Merkel Cell Carcinoma.

480. Resection of local lymph nodes and radiation therapy is used to treat Merkel Cell Carcinoma. It is a very aggressive carcinoma; prognosis is worse than malignant melanoma.

481. The topical antibiotic mafenide acetate can cause metabolic acidosis thorough effect of carbonic anhydrase inhibition. It is used in fresh skin grafts

482. Metastasis is related to motility, transport, arrest and extravasation at end site. "Angiogenic switch" leads to

the growth of blood vessels around the tumor and increases the potential for metastasis.

483. Cathepsin D is used as a prognosticator for breast cancer spread. Its presence increases the risk.

484. Morbid Obesity is associated with sleep apnea, coronary artery disease and diabetes mellitus and osteoarthritis.

485. Consequences of Diabetes Mellitus on the Eye are cumulative over the long run.

Diabetic Retinopathy can be nonproliferative or proliferative.

Normal

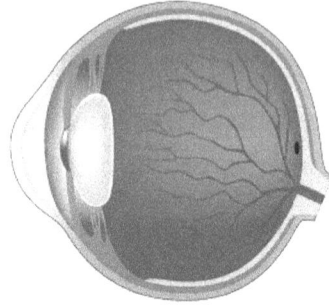

Diabetic Retinopathy

Nonproliferative Retinopathy

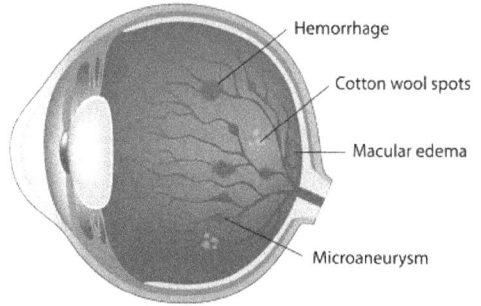

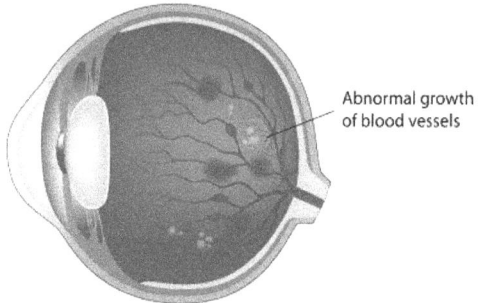

Hemorrhage

Cotton wool spots

Macular edema

Microaneurysm

Proliferative Retinopathy

Abnormal growth of blood vessels

486. History of renal stones, peptic ulcer, and nipple discharge may indicate MEN 1. This is a syndrome of pituitary adenoma, prolactin-secreting adenomas, parathyroid adenomas, pancreatic islet cell tumors – gastrinomas, and insulinomas (The three Ps)

487. MEN 1 can be screened by Gastrin levels, parathyroid hormone (PTH) and prolactin and somatomedin C levels.

488. MEN 2 syndrome is associated with Follicular Thyroid Cancer, Hyperparathyroidism, and Pheochromocytoma.

489. MEN 2 can be screened by PTH, Calcitonin, and Urinary Catecholamines

490. Acute Myocardial Ischemia-related infarction causes coagulative necrosis of the heart muscle.

491. In surviving muscle cells after acute myocardial ischemia, a reversible swelling of the endoplasmic reticulum is seen as a finding.

492. Epstein-Barr virus infection has been associated with the myocarditis and viral cardiomyopathy.

493. There is a high incidence of nasopharyngeal carcinoma in the Chinese.

494. In obstructive jaundice, alkaline phosphatase, GGT (Gamma-glutamyl transferase) and leucine aminopeptidase are elevated.

495. Obstructive Sleep Apnea (OSA) leads to right ventricular failure, hypoxemia, hypercapnia, polycythemia (due to hypoxemia).

496. In OSA, it can lead to cardiac arrhythmia, myocardial infarction, and death

497. Pentalogy of Cantrell is also called thoracoabdominal syndrome. It was characterized in 1958.[2]

A locus at Xq25-26 is cited

 The syndrome has five characteristic findings:

Anterior diaphragmatic hernia

Sternal cleft.

Ectopic Cordis

Omphalocele.

Ventricular septal defect or a diverticulum of the left ventricle.

498. Collagen Type I protein is defective in Osteogenesis Imperfecta

499. The blue sclerae of osteogenesis imperfect is a clue a clue for the existence of the brittle bone disease. The individual may have a history of multiple fractures, may be shorter in height and may have neurological conditions such as communicating hydrocephalus, hearing loss, basilar invagination or seizures. The fractures can cause chronic pain issues and related depression.

500. Acrodermatitis enteropathica is associated with an inability to absorb zinc. This interferes with the ability to form granulation tissue and delays wound healing.

501. Acrodermatitis enteropathica is a rare inherited autosomal recessive disorder that causes problems with zinc absorption leading to a state of zinc deficiency, It is characterized by periorificial and acral dermatitis, alopecia, and diarrhea.

502. The most common organism causing otitis externa is Pseudomonas externa.

503. Rupture of the tympanic membrane in acute otitis media can lead to blood tinged purulent discharge and may accompanied by a relief of pain.

504. Acute Otitis media is linked with conductive hearing loss, not sensory neural hearing loss.

505. Otosclerosis of the bones in the middle ear can lead to a conductive hearing loss.

506. The most common ovarian tumor in children is teratoma.

507. Overfeeding in a critically ill patient can lead to prolonged ventilatory support.

508. Papillary thyroid cancer is most often associated with radiation exposure.

509. A psammoma body is a collection of calcium that can have the appearance of small lumps of sand. These may be found in tumors such as papillary renal cell carcinoma, papillary thyroid carcinoma, micropapillary lung adenocarcinoma, endometrial adenocarcinomas, prolactinomas, meningiomas and others.

510. Pleomorphic Adenoma is the most common salivary gland tumor. It is a benign tumor. It often involves both the parotid glands.

511. Salivary gland malignant mixed tumor is more common in males.

512. When facial nerve is involved in parotid malignancy, there is a facial droop on that side.

513. If there is pain and facial droop associated with a parotid tumor, there is a high chance that it is malignant - mucoepidermoid carcinoma.

514. An abnormal aPTT indicates problems with the intrinsic pathway

515. A patient with prolonged aPTT and deep vein thrombosis should be checked for antiphospholipid syndrome.

516. Antiphospholipid (AN-te-fos-fo-LIP-id) antibody syndrome (APS) is an autoimmune disorder. Autoimmune disorders occur if the body's immune system makes antibodies that attack and damage tissues or cells.

517. Antibodies are a type of protein. They usually help defend the body against infections. In APS, however, the body makes antibodies that mistakenly attack phospholipids—a type of fat.

518. Phospholipids are found in all living cells and cell membranes, including blood cells and the lining of blood vessels.

519. When antibodies attack phospholipids, cells are damaged. This damage causes blood clots to form in the body's arteries and veins.

520. Usually, blood clotting is a normal bodily process. Blood clots help seal small cuts or breaks on blood vessel walls. This prevents you from losing too much blood. In APS, however, too much blood clotting can block blood flow and damage the body's organs.

521. Phaeochromocytoma – has a rule of 10. Ten percent are in children, ten percent are bilateral, ten percent are malignant

522. In Phaeochromocytoma – there may be hypertension, episodic palpitations, headache, sweating whenever the catecholamines are dumped into the blood stream.

523. Polycystic liver disease is often linked to the gene that also causes polycystic kidney disease and intracranial aneurysms.

524. Prune belly syndrome is associated with the lax abdominal wall, dilated ureters, bilateral undescended testis.

525. Prune belly syndrome is characterized by a congenital absence of the abdominal muscles. This leads to a flaccid abdominal wall and prune-like appearance. Most common in females and may be associated with GU abnormalities. It is an X-linked disease.

526. Pseudomembranous enterocolitis is related to the use of antibiotics and overgrowth of Clostridium difficile. Vancomycin and metronidazole can be used to treat it.

527. A C difficile exotoxin assay can help to confirm.

528. Hemorrhagic red infarct can be found with pulmonary embolism

529. In pulmonary sequestration, the blood supply of the lung comes from the aorta

530. Lymphocytes are involved in the donor kidney rejection process

531. Reidel's Thyroiditis; Reidel's Struma may be associated with retroperitoneal fibrosis.

532. Riedel thyroiditis or Riedel's thyroiditis (RT), a chronic inflammatory thyroid disease. It is characterized by the presence of dense fibrosis in the thyroid parenchyma. This fibrotic process can extend beyond the capsule of the thyroid gland.

533. This encroachment of surrounding structures may lead to a change in voice, airway obstruction, hypothyroidism, and hypoparathyroidism. Bronchial obstruction may also lead to stridor.

534. Sacrococcygeal teratomas are benign at birth in 90 percent of the cases but need to be monitored as they can turn malignant. Alpha feto protein (AFP) is a marker that is useful to monitor.

535. A majority of the salivary gland tumors arise in the parotid gland.

536. Salivary gland Warthin's tumor is predominantly found in men

537. Warthin's tumor is a benign cystic tumor of the salivary glands containing lymphocytes and germinal centers (lymph node stroma).

538. Adenocarcinoma accounts for 20 percent of malignant salivary tumors.

539. The treatment of streptococcal pharyngitis prevents rheumatic fever but does not prevent glomerulonephritis or scarlet fever.

540. Sebaceous cysts are a misnomer. They don't contain sebum but keratin.

541. Sepsis can increase metabolic needs/demand by 50 percent

542. ADH is secreted in response to shock to increase volume and it is associated with mesenteric vasoconstriction circulation (to divert blood to more vital areas).

543. Shock following carbon monoxide poisoning is vasodilatory.

544. The most common cause of vasodilatory shock is septic shock.

545. Central Cord Syndrome: Central cord syndrome (CCS) This is a syndrome associated with acute spinal cord injury. In this syndrome, the upper limbs are affected with the loss of motor strength to a greater degree than the lower extremities. There is also dysfunction of the urinary bladder as well as some amount of sensory loss below the level of the injury.

546. Ear discharge and facial palsy indicates vestibular neuronitis associated with cholesteatoma.

547. Bell's palsy signifies facial palsy. It is often caused by a viral infection such as Herpes simplex. It is not related to any aural (ear) discharge.

548. A capillary hemangioma with a port-wine stain on the face may indicate the presence of berry aneurysms.

549. A CT scan of the head is indicated to rule out the presence of berry aneurysms.

550. A cyst near the angle of the mandible may be a branchial type I cyst and will most likely be linked to the external auditory canal.

551. A cyst anterior to the sternocleidomastoid muscle in the neck most likely will be linked to the tonsil pillar on that side. It is related to the second branchial arch.

552. Third branchial clefts linked to the pyriform sinus on that side.

553. Lung cancer is the most common cancer in the world followed by breast cancer and then stomach cancer.

554. Atypical lobular hyperplasia increases the risk of breast cancer in women.

555. Germline mutations in the following genes are associated with higher risk for breast cancer BRCA1, BRCA2 and P 53

556. P 53 has also been linked to other cancers other than breast cancer such as brain cancer, sarcomas, adrenocortical carcinomas, leukemia.

557. The risk of ovarian cancer is also increased with BRCA1 and to a smaller degree with BRCA2.

558. Bronchiectasis is linked to infection by non-tubercular mycobacteria infection. Bronchiectasis is also linked to cystic fibrosis and Kartagener syndrome.

559. Kartagener syndrome is associated with problems of motility of the cilia and may also lead to infertility.

560. The affinity of carbon monoxide is 200 to 250 times greater for hemoglobin and then the affinity of oxygen for hemoglobin.

561. Chronic granulomatous disease is linked with recurrent infections in different systems. It is related to a deficiency of NADPH oxidase activity. Cyanide poisoning can occur from smoke inhalation.

562. Hydroxycobalamin is used as an antidote for such situations of cyanide poisoning.

Cystic Fibrosis

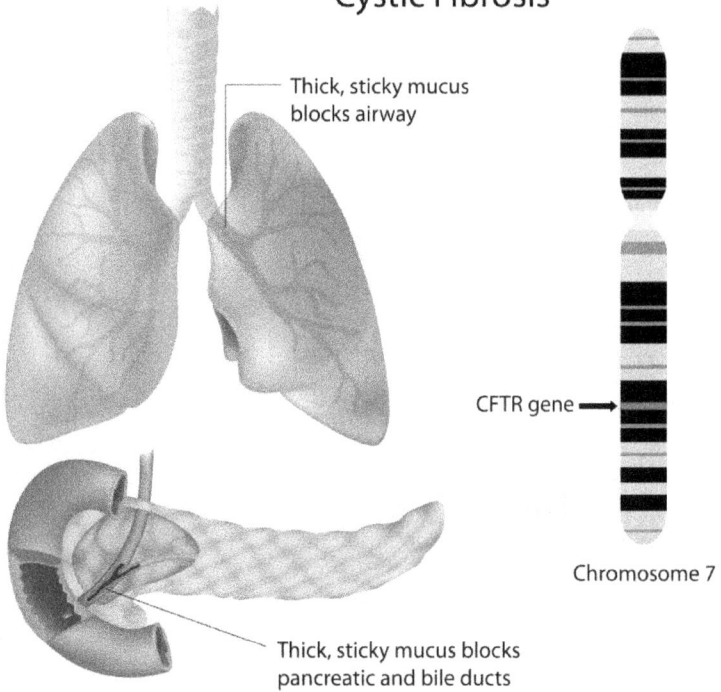

Thick, sticky mucus blocks airway

CFTR gene →

Chromosome 7

Thick, sticky mucus blocks pancreatic and bile ducts

563.

564. The nitroblue tetrazolium reduction test is used for diagnosing CGD.

565. Hepatocellular carcinoma can lead to gynecomastia due to the increased production of estrogen.

566. The hallmark of Cri-du-Chat syndrome is a high-pitched catlike crying and severe mental retardation.

567. The Cri- du- Chat syndrome is associated with an anomaly in chromosome 5p-

568. The most common cause for Cushing's disease is a pituitary adenoma that produces too much ACTH.

569. The 24 hour urinary 17OH (17 hydroxy) corticosteroid level is the most sensitive test to detect hypercortisolism.

570. A low dose dexamethasone suppression test can be used to confirm hypercortisolism.

571. The cytochrome P4 50 system breaks down compound by oxidation-reduction and hydrolysis. Not by conjugation.

572. Hypokalemia causes decreased deep tendon reflexes.

573. Hypomagnesaemia and hypocalcemia cause an increase in deep tendon reflexes making them more brisk and pronounced.

574. Hypoglycemia does not affect the deep tendon reflexes.

575. Desmoid tumors of the chest wall are linked to the presence of adenomatous polyposis coli (APC).

576. Gardner Syndrome is a syndrome that is also known as familial adenomatous polyposis. In this syndrome, there are multiple benign tumors in different body parts. This may include sebaceous cysts, epidermoid cysts, fibromas, osteomas and desmoid tumors.

577. Diabetes insipidus is suggested by the presence of a dilute urine (less than 300 osmol/L) and hypernatremia. DDAVP is helpful. Brain tumors, injury can cause central DI.

578. Lithium can cause nephrogenic diabetes insipidus. DDAVP does not help this.

579. Potassium-sparing diuretics such as amiloride and triamterene are used sometimes to help with lithium-induced diabetes insipidus. Sometimes the lithium has to be discontinued, and other agents such as divalproic acid have to be used to control symptoms of bipolar disorder- for which lithium is prescribed.

580. If the serum sodium is elevated, think about Cushing's syndrome. This syndrome includes an excess production of both corticosteroids and mineralocorticoids such as aldosterone which causes the increased sodium retention and hypernatremia.

581. Conn's syndrome is a syndrome of only primary hyperaldosteronism. It is associated with high blood pressure, hypernatremia, and hypokalemia. Does not affect the glucocorticoids such as cortisol.

582. Conn's syndrome is inherited hyperaldosteronism. The excess of aldosterone leads to Na (sodium) retention, k (potassium) loss (leading to hypokalemia) and metabolic alkalosis (bicarbonate reabsorbed when k excreted).

583. The Glasgow coma scale is a scale to describe the level of consciousness after a traumatic brain injury. It cannot be lower than three. The lower the number the worst and deeper the coma is. Severe is anything below 8 and it goes up by 3's.

    3-8 Severe Coma

    9-12 moderate coma

    13 to 15 mild coma

584. In diabetes, it is the neuropathy with a decrease in sensation to pain that leads to the diabetic foot ulcers. This is why diabetics are always advised to wear shoes so that they don't accidentally injure their feet without even knowing it.

585. Normal anion gap acidosis is related to diarrhea or G.I. losses. The loss of bicarbonate leads to the acidosis.

586. Patients with down syndrome are at increased risk for developing lymphoblastic leukemia.

587. Approximately 1/3 of patients with down syndrome are also born with duodenal atresia.

588. In duodenal atresia, a part of the duodenum does not develop properly and delays the passage of gastric contents. Surgery is corrective.

Symptoms of duodenal atresia include:

589. Upper abdominal swelling (sometimes)

590. Early vomiting of large amounts, which may be greenish (because of bile being vomited)

591. Continued vomiting even when infant has not been fed for several hours

592. The way to differentiate congenital pyloric stenosis and duodenal atresia is to note the following.
In Duodenal atresia, bile is present in vomitus
Down's syndrome is more likely to associated with duodenal atresia
Polyhydramnios is often seen in mother who bears the child with duodenal atresia.

593. Pyloric stenosis is caused by hypertrophy of the muscles surrounding the opening of the stomach into the duodenum. This condition leads to projectile vomiting. The vomit does not contain bile.

594. Down syndrome patient should also be checked for any cardiac anomalies.

595. The Ehler Danlos is an autosomal dominant syndrome marked by a defect in collagen formation. The skin is stretchy. There may be arteriovenous fistulas.

596. Timely treatment of strep throat (is caused by Group A beta-hemolytic streptococci) can prevent Rheumatic fever

597. In Factor V Leiden disease, there is an inability to inactivate Factor V and this leads to increased thrombosis tendency

598. Factor XIII deficiency leads to delayed bleeding after injury or surgery

599. Fatty liver disease is marked by the accumulation of triglycerides within hepatocytes.

Healthy liver   ## Fatty liver

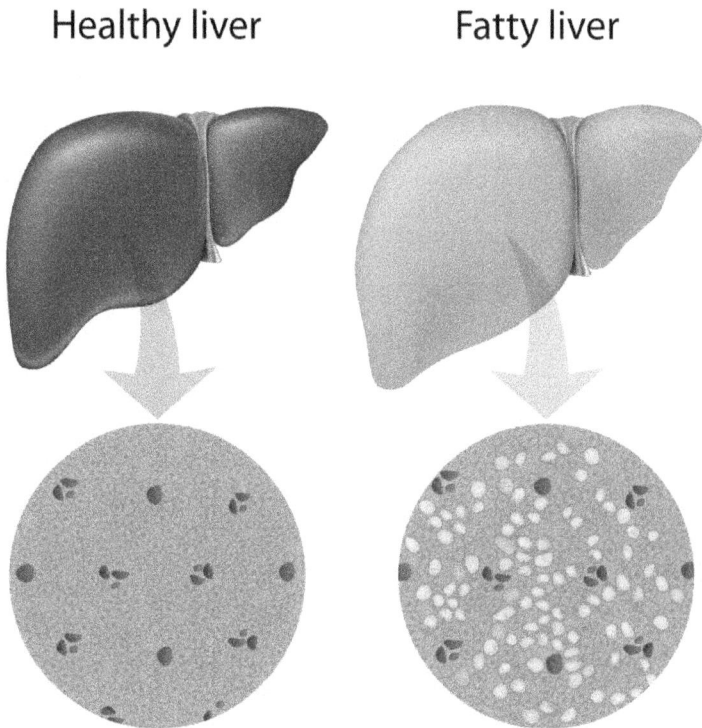

600. The absence of breast is rare and is associated with Poland syndrome.

601. In Fleischer's syndrome, there is displacement of the nipples and hypoplasia or underdevelopment of the kidneys.

602. And Klinefelter syndrome, there is an XXY chromosome pattern. It is associated with gynecomastia,

hypogonadism, and azoospermia. There is also a higher risk of breast cancer in patients with XXY syndrome.

603. Focal nodular hyperplasia is benign and associated with a stellate scar and Kupfer cells.

604. In hepatic adenomas, there are Kupfer cells.

605. Follicular thyroid cancer is spread through the bloodstream to the bone. This type of cancer may be more common in areas that are deficient in iodine.

606. Papillary thyroid cancer spreads through the lymphatic system.

607. Formic acid exposure has been associated with hemolysis and hemoglobinuria.

608. Gastric infection with Helicobacter pylori he has been associated with duodenal ulcers, gastric ulcers, gastric cancer and chronic gastritis.

609. Gout is due to under excretion or overproduction of uric acid. Treatment is with Finnegan is allopurinol.

610. Following surgery on the parotid glands, there may occur the phenomenon of gustatory sweating, In this, there may be a crossover linkage during surgery and healing between the auriculotemporal nerve and the sympathetic nerves of the skin. When there is something tasty (gustatory stimulus), the parotid gland nerves are stimulated, and this leads to stimulation of

the skin sympathetic nerves that cause sweating of the skin in that area of distribution.

611. In hepatocellular carcinoma, there is increased estrogen production and development of breasts or gynecomastia.

612. In Hashimoto's thyroiditis, there may be a diffuse tenderness of the thyroid gland, hypothyroidism, and weight gain.

613. Hashimoto's thyroiditis occurs in a middle-aged woman and is the most common form of thyroiditis.

614. And chronic heart failure, there is leakage of red blood cells through the capillaries of the congested lungs. These red blood cells are ingested by WBC's, and their hemosiderin is evident on examination. These hemosiderin laden white blood cells are called heart failure cells. Below is a picture. The dark brown cells are the heart failure cells in the alveoli.

615. Heat shock proteins are formed under conditions of stress such as ischemia, trauma, burns, and radiation exposure to heavy metals. They regulate the inflammatory response and the immune response in order to minimize damage to the tissues. They can be pro-or anti-inflammatory at different junctures of the response to the trauma.

616. The most common cause of congenital hemolytic anemia is a pyruvate kinase deficiency.

617. Hemophilia C is caused by a deficiency of factor XI. It is more common in Ashkenazi Jews.

618. A patient with partial albinism and a bleeding disorder may have dense granule deficiency disease. Also called Hermansky Pudlak syndrome.

619. Heparin-induced thrombocytopenia or HIT is caused by the formation of an antibody to PF4 (platelet factor 4). This antibody interferes with platelet activation and leads to thrombosis formation.

620. H I T should be suspected if the platelet count falls below hundred thousand or decreases by 50% in the patient started on heparin.

621. Hepatic Adenoma is associated with the use of oral contraceptives. It may have a tendency to bleed or become malignant.

622. Hepatocellular carcinoma is associated with infection by hepatitis B, hepatitis C and with alcoholic cirrhosis.

623. Exposure to Aflatoxin is associated with liver cancer.

624. Aflatoxin: This is a toxin related to the mold Aspergillus. It can lead to hepatitis and liver cancer.

625. The fungi that produce aflatoxin grow on crops such as peanuts (especially) and wheat, corn, beans and rice.

626. Aflatoxin is a problem particularly in undeveloped and developing countries such as China.

627. Fibrolamellar liver cancer tends to be more common in females. There is type of cancer tends to occur in younger individuals less than 35 and is characterized by sheets of hepatocytes that are well differentiated and separated by a fibrous tissue. It is, therefore, resectable and has a better prognosis.

     It is not associated with hepatitis B, cirrhosis or elevated AFP levels.

628. Standard hepatocellular liver cancer tends to be more common in males.

629. Neither tumor is associated with hepatitis A.

630. Marked elevation of AFP [more than 400 ng/mL] is associated with hepatocellular carcinoma and teratocarcinoma.

631. Teratocarcinoma is a germ cell tumor of the testis.

632. A germ cell tumor occurs inside the gonads i.e., the testis or the ovary. They may be benign or malignant. Sometimes germ cells may be found outside the gonads due to developmental anomalies.

633. Individuals with Hirschsprung disease have mutations has several levels. This includes GDNF, Ret and it's coreceptor Gfra-1.

634. Hirschsprung's disease (HSCR) (congenital megacolon) is marked the absence of nerve cells in the myenteric plexus between the smooth muscles of the large colon. This leads impaired peristalsis and severe constipation. Bowel obstruction can occur requiring medical intervention.

635. Hidradenitis Suppurativa is an acneiform infection involving the apocrine glands in several areas.

636. The apocrine gland is a type of sweat gland.

637. The skin has two types of sweat glands: the eccrine glands and apocrine glands. Eccrine glands open directly onto the surface of the skin. Apocrine glands develop in areas abundant in hair follicles, such as the groin and armpits. They empty into the hair follicle just before it opens to the skin surface.

638. When the temperature in the environment rises or if there is excessive physical exertion, the eccrine glands secrete sweat onto the surface of the skin, where it cools the body by evaporation. This fluid is composed mainly of water and salt.

639. Apocrine glands produce a milky fluid that is secreted periodically due to different stimuli. This fluid is odorless until it combines with bacteria found on the skin.

640. Homogentisic oxidase deficiency is associated with urine that turns dark on standing. It is associated with blue, black pigmentation of the sclerae and arthritis.

641. Hyperaldosteronism is also called Conn's syndrome. In primary hyperaldosteronism, the plasma renin levels are suppressed. In secondary hyperaldosteronism (due to a need to raise blood pressure due to volume loss or other factors), the plasma renin level will be high. So plasma renin level differentiates primary and secondary type

642. Chromium deficiency may be associated with glucose intolerance and a rash on the hands. This type of deficiency is more likely to develop the in patients that are fed by TPN. Other micronutrient deficiencies may also develop.

643. TPN stands for total parenteral nutrition is a the nutritional support offered through intravenous infusions. This is usually a short-term measure usually provided when patients are unable to take nutrition by mouth. Some patients are given TPN for long periods such as when they are in a coma.

644. Risk factors for hyperparathyroidism are as follows: postmenopausal female, history of radiation, family

history of multiple endocrine Neoplasia type I syndrome.

645. Symptoms of hyperparathyroidism owner moans (depression), groans (myalgia, pain) and stones (kidney stones-nephrolithiasis).

646. Carpopedal spasm is not found in hyperparathyroidism because the calcium level is high. Carpopedal spasm occurs when the calcium level is low due to *hypo*parathyroidism.

647. Marfan's syndrome- proteins affected are fibrillin, elastin; mutation is on Chromosome 15 called FBNI mutation

648. The familial hypocalciuric syndrome is a rare genetic cause of hypercalcemia. Not enough calcium is excreted in urine so the plasma Ca level is elevated.

649. Parathyroid adenoma is the usual suspect in the cause of hypercalcemia.

650. Milk-alkali syndrome is elevated calcium due to excessive intake of calcium. Can occur if someone takes a lot of antacid that has antacid such as calcium hydroxide, or is trying to treat osteoporosis with supplemental calcium.

651. Someone with cirrhosis and ascites can develop spontaneous peritonitis due to an infection that can present as abdominal pain. Fever may not be present; antibiotic cefotaxime recommended until culture results available.

652. Tourette's disorder can present with vocal and motor tics and is not a seizure disorder. Treatment is dopamine blocker such as pimozide or haloperidol.

653. Ventriculoseptal defect is the most common congenital heart defect. Most close soon after birth. May be associated with Down's syndrome.

654. Alcohol withdrawal may present as confusion, elevated vitals within 24 to 48 hours of last alcohol containing drink. Keep this differential high in someone with a history of alcoholism disclosed or undisclosed. Alcohol-dependent patients undergoing surgical procedures may run into alcohol withdrawal problems such as elevated vital signs or frank delirium if they have a hidden or minimized their alcohol dependence problems. The key to preventing complications is to get collateral history and provide treatment for withdrawal with thiamine, and benzodiazepines in adequate doses to control and suppress the withdrawal symptoms.

655. Treatment of alcohol dependence is Thiamine 100 mg im or iv, then po benzodiazepines to control the

withdrawal symptoms. Adequate treatment of withdrawal and prevention of delirium tremens is very important. In addition to initial IM or IV thiamine, supplementation with Folic acid, oral thiamine, multivitamin and magnesium (if low) is recommended in the detox regimen. Full detox may take up to a week.

656. There is a significant mortality with untreated delirium tremens (DT). The mortality rates vary from 5 to 15%. If DT develops, the care of the patient should be transferred to the ICU.

657. Oxygen-hemoglobin dissociation curve- shift to left indicates high affinity for oxygen, shift to right means lower affinity for oxygen.

658. Acidosis can cause the shift to the right.

659. Bacterial vaginosis caused by Gardnerella vaginalis causes gray fishy smell discharge

660. Trichomonas vaginalis causes greenish foul smelling discharge

661. Chlamydia infection by Chlamydia trachomatis is the most common sexually transmitted disease in the US. Can cause cervicitis, urethritis, salpingitis, arthritis, and conjunctivitis. Cervical discharge is purulent, cervical motion tenderness is present and is called Chandelier sign.

662. Candidiasis- whitish cotton cheese type discharge

663. Genital Herpes- painful shallow ulcers on genitalia surface, fever, headache, muscle pain associated

664. Gonorrhea associated with purulent discharge

665. Intracellular diplococci Neisseria gonorrhoeae causes gonorrhea.

666. In psychiatric patients acute neck stiffness is caused by antipsychotics such as haloperidol, fluphenazine-treatment is with benztropine 2 mgs IM or PO, diphenhydramine (Benadryl) 50 mgs IM or PO can also be used.

667. Akathisia is a sense of restlessness caused by antipsychotics – treatment is with benztropine and or beta blockers such as propranolol. Switching to a less potent dopamine receptor blocking antipsychotic may also help.

668. Tardive Dyskinesia is a syndrome of involuntary movements associated with the long-term use of antipsychotics.

669. Dual-energy xray absorptiometry is the procedure used to detect osteoporosis. Osteoporosis is defined as a bone density below 2.5 standard deviations of a young adult.

670. Pulmonary hypertension is when the pulmonary artery pressure is greater than the 70% of the systemic pressure. May present as dyspnea in a young pregnant

mother. The risk to mother is significant if present. It may be a reason for elective medical termination of pregnancy- MTP or therapeutic abortion to save the mother's life.

671. Trick Question: A Brain biopsy is the <u>most accurate test to confirm</u> a brain tumor. An MRI or CT scan may be ordered however as an initial screen.

672. A clue from liver enzymes: AST is higher than ALT in alcoholics. <u>S</u> in AST for <u>S</u>pirit is a clue. Alcoholic cardiomyopathy can cause congestive heart failure.

673. HIV drug zidovudine causes mitochondrial changes in cells.

674. HIV, Simvastatin, Alcohol, cocaine abuse can cause myositis.

675. Takayasu's arteritis is found in young Asian females is an arteritis that can cause low blood pressure, muscle pains. Wt loss is common

676. Acute tubular necrosis is the result of volume loss. Rise in blood urea nitrogen (azotemia), Cr, Muddy brown epithelial casts and granular casts found in urine, proteinuria

677. humpy lumpy deposits in acute glomerulonephritis. Type III reaction.

678. Interstitial nephritis is reaction around tubules caused by drugs, infection. Eosinophilia may occur.

679. Hypothyroidism associated with wt gain, menstrual irregularities, galactorrhea, sensitivity to cold, constipation, dry skin, slowed tendon reflexes

680. In aortic valve stenosis, surgery for aortic valve replacement is indicated if the separation of valves is less than 8 mm. This is checked by echocardiography. This surgery is indicated if the patient is symptomatic (dyspnea, dizziness or chest pain). Coronary artery bypass surgery if planned is also an indication to have the valve also replaced.

681. For influenza, amantadine and zanamivir are helpful if offered in the first 48 hours of the onset of flu symptoms.

682. ACE inhibitors such as Lisinopril or ARB's such as losartan are first line agents for many individuals with hypertension due to the protective effect provided to the kidneys for nephropathy related to hypertension.

683. ARB's have the advantage of not causing the side effect of cough that can occur with some ACE inhibitors.

684. Doxazosin is a smooth muscle relaxer (selective alpha 1 blocker) that is used for htn in patients that also have prostatic hypertrophy (BPH) as it helps both the conditions. Dizziness upon arising is a risk with alpha blockers. This is called orthostatic hypotension (blood

pools in the lower legs upon arising leading to decrease in blood pressure and dizziness. With time, body makes adjustments)

685. Hydralazine is also a smooth muscle blocker but is not used much due to side effect of causing SLE-like syndrome.

686. Colonoscopy is recommended for all persons after 50 as screening for CA colon and then every 10 years if no polyps.

687. A person is deemed competent and has the right to refuse medication and care. Only a court of law can deem a patient to be incompetent and may appoint a conservator.

688. Pain in the flank, costovertebral tenderness and fever can have a high chance of being acute pyelonephritis. Get UA, culture, treat as indicated by sensitivity.

689. In AIDS, the most useful test to measure progress of HIV infection is HIV RT PCR . A viral load of 750,000 or more is not good. CD 4 is often the wrong answer for a question about measuring HIV progression.

690. CD 4 count is useful once someone already has AIDS to decide on what prophylactic treatment to prevent infection is recommended.

691. Brief psychotic disorder lasts from a day to less than a month. It is induced in some people by acute stressors.

692. A child with hematuria, deafness, eye problems and family member with similar problems may have Alport's syndrome – x linked recessive.

693. In Wilm's tumor caused by chromosome 11 disorder, children age 2-4 years of age present with a flank mass that may be palpable. Hematuria may also be present.

694. Wilms tumor is sometimes associated with aniridia (absence of the iris), genitourinary symptoms and retardation. This is called the WAGRS complex.

695. C-11 hydroxylase deficiency can present as precocious early puberty, hypertension and aggressive behaviors due to high testosterone levels from stimulation of adrenal glands.

696. C21 hydroxylase also leads to increased testosterone levels, and low cortisol and aldosterone levels. It leads to low blood pressure due to low aldosterone.

697. 17 hydroxylase deficiency leads to delayed puberty.

698. Picture of Down's baby or child (upturned outer canthus of eyes)- most common associated cardiac defect is AV septal defect.

699. Turner's syndrome- short webbed neck 45xo, associated with coarctation of the aorta and bicuspid aortic valve.

700. 22q11 syndrome (DiGeorge Syndrome) associated with Tetralogy of Fallot and persistent truncus arteriosus.

701. Infants of Diabetic mother have a higher risk for transposition of great vessels

702. Fungal infection of toes causes discoloration, hyphae seen under microscope

703. Hunter Syndrome is x linked recessive lysosome storage disease. The syndrome is marked by some characteristic features such as a large head, hepatosplenomegaly. The enzyme, iduronate-2-sulfatase is noted to be deficient. Other associated features include diarrhea, mental retardation, and aggressive behavior.

704. Topical radiation therapy is the treatment of choice for first stage vaginal cancer.

705. More infiltrative vaginal cancer may need surgery and radiation. Chemotherapy is used after surgery as well. Hormonal treatment is not indicated.

706. Mallory-Weis tears occur in the lower esophagus after a prolonged bout of vomiting.

707. The most common age of onset of eczema is 1-2 years of age. Skin is dry and scaly.

708. Seborrheic dermatitis, dandruff can affect immunocompromised individuals more often

709. Scabies is caused by mite Sarcoptes Scabei- very itchy at night, mite burrows under the skin.

710. Ankylosing spondylitis causes stiffness and pain in lower back. Uveitis and photosensitivity may be associated with about 40 percent of cases. HLA B-27 associated.

711. Case-Control Study is a retrospective study looking at factors associated with a certain disease and a group of individuals without the disease.

712. Alcoholics can develop B3 (niacin) deficiency (Pellagra) and related problems of diarrhea, dementia, and dermatitis. Dermatitis around the neck is called pellagra casal necklace

713. Vitamin A deficiency is associated with night blindness.

714. Vitamin C deficiency causes scurvy

715. Vit D deficiency causes rickets in children and osteomalacia in adults.

716. Deficiency of folic acid in pregnant mothers can cause neural tube defects in the infant.

717. Projection: The motives that lie within oneself are attributed to others.

718. Transference- The patient projects feelings from a significant other towards the doctor

719. Countertransference: The doctor projects feelings from another significant relationship to the patient. The doctor must never act on any unusual feelings of anger or liking for the patient. Remain professional and cordial. Such patients should be transferred to a colleague if there are difficulties dealing with the patient due to transference or countertransference.

720. Sublimation is transforming a negative emotional state into a positive one such as humor or altruistic or charitable works.

721. Reaction formation: The individual in this type of defensive psychological reaction generates behaviors opposite to the feelings to what he or she feels. Libidinous feelings thus as an example may be acted in a manner opposite to what would be expected of the person becoming a priest or a nun. A corrupt politician may campaign against corruption is another type reaction formation.

722. Choriocarcinoma is a cancer of the placenta. HCG is elevated. May spread to lungs. Symptoms may include abnormal vaginal bleeding after the recent birth of a child.

723. A woman of child bearing age has cramping and vaginal bleeding, think of ectopic pregnancy or miscarriage.

724. Next step is to get a pregnancy test. Next step is a trick question. It is the next logical step; they are not asking for the most important test. Ultrasonography may be very important and give vital information.

725. Testicular torsion may present with acute abdominal pain and is a surgical emergency.

726. N acetyl cysteine is the treatment of choice for an overdose of acetaminophen.

727. Pyridoxine is drug of choice for INH poisoning

728. Fomepizole is drug of choice for methanol poisoning or ethylene glycol poisoning.

729. Calcium gluconate for hydrofluoric acid toxicity

730. Next step is often different from the diagnostic step, read the question carefully.

731. For an elderly person who is found wandering in the neighborhood in a confused state and there are no medical problems: The next step would be to do a mini mental status exam.

732. Alexia is the loss of ability to read. It is related to strokes in the area of the posterior cerebral artery.

733. Apraxia is the loss of ability to do simple tasks. Posterior parietal cortex involved.

734. Aphasia is the result of damage to temporal speech area. Anterior damage associated with Broca's aphasia-lack of ability to speak

Wernicke's aphasia is due to damage to posterior temporal area. Person can speak but cannot understand spoken speech

735. Agnosia is the inability to recognize common objects-due to damage to the occipitotemporal border area.

736. Some jaundice in newborn due to elevated unconjugated bilirubin may be normal. Light therapy is helpful.

737. Aminoglycosides are gentamycin, streptomycin, amikacin, tobramycin

738. Side effects of Aminoglycosides can be remembered with phrase : NO NEED OF TOXINS

    Stands for: Nephrotoxicity, Neuromuscular blockade, Ototoxicity, and Teratogen

739. Menetrier Disease- increased folds in stomach lining- protein loss occurs- decreased osmotic pressure- leads to edema

740. Herpes Simplex Virus associated with "punched out ulcers" in lower esophagus

741. Vinyl Chloride causes angiosarcoma of liver. Used in rubber industry

742. Location and size of carcinoid tumor predicts spread

743. Nonkeratinizing squamous epithelium found in esophagus

744. Nonciliated columnar epithelium found in Barret's esophagus

745. Gastric tissue can be found in ectopic places and lead to ulcers

746. Omphalocele is an umbilical hernia

747. Meconium ileus is thick mucus in small intestine lumen of infant secreted by pancreas- found with cystic fibrosis- may lead to perforation

748. Primary Sclerosing Cholangitis- fever, pain, right upper quadrant pain- association with ulcerative colitis

749. Wilson's Disease- copper metabolism problem- increased urinary copper, increased copper in the liver, decreased ceruloplasmin, and Kayser-Fleischer Rings in the cornea. Deposition of copper in the basal ganglia may cause parkinsonian symptoms

750. Celiac Disease is related to gluten intolerance and damage is most evident in the proximal earlier part of the small intestine.

751. Reye Syndrome- caused by the use of aspirin for fever with viral infections- associated with adverse effects on liver and brain.

752. Scleroderma (Progressive Systemic Sclerosis) is associated with difficulty swallowing.

753. Plummer-Vinson Syndrome- is related to iron deficiency, atrophic glossitis, esophageal webs in upper esophagus and difficulty swallowing.

754. Zenker Diverticulum- a small diverticulum in upper esophagus

755. Oral cancer commonly found in floor of mouth, tip of tongue- initial change may be a whitish change- leukoplakia

756. Mallory-Weiss tears in lower esophagus are tears associated with severe vomiting.

757. Hematemesis or vomiting of blood without prior vomiting more likely be due to esophageal varices.

758. Pancreatic Cancer can present with symptoms of depression, palpable gallbladder, vague mid abdominal pain, and jaundice.

759. S-100 is marker for Melanoma tumor

760. Alpha-fetoprotein and alpha1 antitrypsin are markers for hepatocellular carcinoma

761. PSA and Prostatic Acid Phosphatase is a marker for Prostate Cancer (Prostatic Carcinoma)

762. CA125 is marker for serous cystadenocarcinoma of the ovary

763. CEA and Bombesin are markers for Gastric Adenocarcinoma

764. Leukoplakia are whitish plaques in mouth with 5 % chance of turning into cancer

765. Melanosis Coli- pigmentation of colon associated with laxative use

766. Lymph nodes from penis, vagina, drain to medial superficial inguinal lymph nodes

767. Coloboma is defect in the midline of the eye

768. Patau Syndrome is Trisomy 13, narrowing of nasal passages, small head, heart defects, defects of ear, coloboma

769. VATER Syndrome is associated with anal atresia, esophageal atresia, vertebral, radial and kidney abnormalities

770. Pancreatic Adenocarcinoma prognosis is dismal (2.5% survival at five years)

771. Esophagus Adenocarcinoma survival rate is also low -10 % survival at five years

772. Primary Biliary Cirrhosis associated with the destruction of medium sized hepatic ducts, increased alkaline phosphatase and increased conjugated bilirubin levels.

773. Budd-Chiari Syndrome associated with occlusion of inferior vena cava or renal vein- liver is congested enlarged, back log can lead to ascites- polycythemia vera, pregnancy, pregnancy a risk factor.

774. PiZZ allele is a variant of alpha1antitrypsin- it is an ineffective variant, leads to alpha1antitrypsin deficiency syndrome.

775. Biliary Stones- can be cholesterol (more in females), brown (calcium variant), and black (calcium and unconjugated bilirubin). The calcium stones are detectable on x-ray.

776. Mucin glycoproteins provide the scaffolding for the stones

777. Acute Hemorrhagic Pancreatitis can cause bleeding, severe pain, necrosis, vomiting, shock related to volume loss due to a massive release of pancreatic enzymes.

778. So if an alcoholic presents with pain vomiting, shock, think of acute hemorrhagic pancreatitis.

779. A man with polycythemia vera presents with hepatomegaly, ascites- think of Budd-Chiari syndrome (syndrome of Inferior vena cava or portal vein obstruction due to blood clot)

780. Giardia Lamblia is the most common intestinal pathogen. May look like a mask.

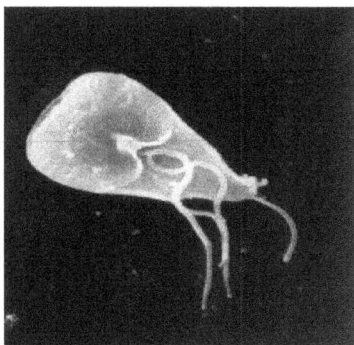

781.

Credit: CDC: http://phil.cdc.gov/phil/

782. Entamoeba Histolytica- is another pathogen that affects the liver and large colon. Very common in India, Asia- treated with metronidazole

783. Naegleria Fowleri causes meningoencephalitis

784. Trichomonas Vaginalis causes vaginitis- most common cause

785. Fat Necrosis- acute pancreatitis releases lipase, this acts on mesenteric fat, releases fats which combine with calcium to form soap -whitish soap deposits on areas of necrosis in the pancreas

786. Shatzki rings are found in the lower esophagus

787. Intussusception occurs between 5 to 10 months of age

788. Congenital pyloric stenosis presents earlier between 2 to 4 weeks

789. Meckel's diverticulum- is due to failure of vitelline duct to atrophy

790. Allantois becomes umbilical cord and placenta

791. Reiter's Syndrome – can't pee (urethritis), can't see (uveitis), can't climb a tree (arthritis)

792. Sjogren's Syndrome- dry eyes due to failure of lacrimal glands- attacked by autoantibody, also has dry mouth and arthritis

793. Hydatid Cyst caused by Echinococcus and rupture of the cyst can lead to shock.

794. Stone in bile duct causes conjugated bilirubin not to go into circulation and this elevated bilirubin get excreted in urine which turns darker. The stool becomes paler, clay-colored due to lack of dark yellow bilirubin. Bilirubin is not present for bacteria in gut to convert to urobilinogen so the urobilinogen levels in circulation and in urine will decrease. A low urobilinogen level in urine therefore indicates possible gallbladder obstruction by stone or carcinoma of head of pancreas that constricts the bile duct and reduces or stops flow of bile.

795. Choledocholithiasis- means stone in the bile duct

796. Antibiotic Clindamycin poses a high risk for overgrowth of Clostridium difficile that cause life threatening necrotizing enterocolitis.

797. Zollinger-Ellison Syndrome causes increased HCl production- ulcers in duodenum more likely than stomach

798. Apoprotein CII turns on lipase in chylomicrons. Lack of it is cause of primary hyperlipidemia.

799. Secretin test for Zollinger-Ellison Syndrome. Injection of secretin causes an abnormal rise in Gastrin.

800. The cancers of intestinal lymphoma and breast cancer are associated with the presence of celiac disease.

801. Type A Gastritis is in Fundus- Upper part of stomach

802. Type B Gastritis is in Antrum- Lower part of stomach

803. Charcot's Triad is marked by Fever, Jaundice, RUQ pain associated with infection, inflammation of the biliary tree proximal to a bile duct obstruction.

804. Dronabinol (Marinol) is a cannabinoid used for the treatment of nausea, vomiting in cancer.

805. Compazine (prochlorperazine) is used for nausea vomiting, works by dopamine receptor blocking effect in the chemoreceptor trigger zone in the floor of the fourth ventricle.

806. Helicobacter pylori associated with duodenal ulcers. Treated with PPI (omeprazole, lansoprazole), and antibiotics (clarithromycin and either metronidazole or amoxicillin)

807. Tegaserod (Zelnorm) stimulates peristalsis and helps with constipation in patients with IBS or due to other causes.

808. Misoprostol stimulates prostaglandin E1 – leads to decreased acid production, greater mucus production

809. Megestrol (Megace), a synthetic oral progestin is used to stimulate appetite in patients with AIDS.

810. Orlistat inactivates lipase that digests lipids

811. For bleeding esophageal varices - Octreotide is used to decrease blood flow to portal circulation.

812. Octreotide is also used to inhibit hormone release from carcinoid tumors.

813. Metoclopramide is dopamine antagonist that increases gastric emptying in gastric paresis. Also, can be used as an antiemetic. Associated with prolonged QTc sometimes with higher doses of metoclopramide.

814. Ursodiol is used to dissolve cholesterol gall stones

815. Docusate works as a laxative by decreasing surface tension at the oil-water interface of the feces allowing more water in the feces. Water intake should, therefore, be encouraged

816. Bulk-forming laxatives such as psyllium and methylcellulose absorb water but are not themselves absorbed and increase in bulk and stimulate peristalsis.

817. Castor oil, senna, and bisacodyl are stimulant laxatives

818. Mineral oil and glycerin are laxatives that coat feces and prevent water loss act as lubricants in the passage of the stools.

819. Sulfasalazine is used to treat mild to moderate ulcerative colitis

820. The chemoreceptor trigger zone is located on the floor of the fourth ventricle. It has dopamine D2 receptors – blocked by traditional antipsychotics such as Compazine and HT3 receptors- blocked by Ondansetron for the control of nausea.

821. Sucralfate is a basic aluminum salt that binds to an ulcer and coats it. Used to treat peptic ulcers.

822. Cimetidine is an H2 blocker used for hyperacidity but is not used much because it is a P450 inhibitor and can inhibit the metabolism of other drugs such as warfarin.

823. Meperidine also known as pethidine is the best analgesic when there is pain due to cholecystitis as it does not cause a constriction of the sphincter of Oddi that surrounds the bile duct as it empties into the small intestine. Opiates such as morphine can cause the sphincter to constrict. The constriction of the sphincter can cause the blockage of the bile duct to worsen and thus worsen the disease process.

824. Cysticerci from pig tapeworm tend to infest the brain and muscles

825. Schistosomiasis tends to involve the urinary bladder.

826. Petechial rashes, jaundice, hepatosplenomegaly, and sensorineural hearing loss is associated with congenital CMV infection

827. Rubivirus causes rubella (German measles) and can cause cardiovascular defects in babies born to mothers infected during pregnancy.

828. Toxoplasma Gondi is associated with chorioretinitis, hydrocephalus, and intracranial calcifications

829. Congenital syphilis (Treponema Pallidum) is associated with hearing loss, Hutchinson teeth, rash on palms and soles of feet

830. Antigenic shift (sudden change) and not antigenic drift is associated with outbreaks of Influenza virus epidemics

831. Coxsackievirus is a picornavirus, the smallest of the RNA viruses but causes big problems with myocarditis. They are positive, <u>single-stranded, naked, icosahedral</u> RNA viruses.

An **ICOSAHEDRON** is composed of 20 facets, each an equilateral triangle

832. The most common causes of urethritis in males are Chlamydia trachomatis and Neisseria gonorrhoeae.

833. Treatment for Chlamydia trachomatis is Azithromycin.

834. Treatment for N gonorrhea is Ceftriaxone

835. Fluconazole is an antifungal agent effective for infections by fungi such candida albicans.

836. Penicillin is effective for syphilis

837. Vancomycin is for treatment resistant S Aureus and for Clostridium difficile

838. Campylobacter jejuni, a comma-shaped, oxidase-positive, gram-negative bacterium can cause gastroenteritis with bloody diarrhea and has been

associated with Guillan Barre syndrome through an immune mediated interaction with peripheral nerves.

839. Pseudomonas aeruginosa can cause otitis externa, urinary tract infection, pneumonia, and sepsis in some hosts with immunocompromised status.

840. Acid-fast bacilli such as Mycobacterium tuberculosis cause TB. Infection of the bone by this organism is known as Pott's disease. This often presents in the vertebrae and can lead to the hunchback or gibbus presentation.

841. Salmonella osteomyelitis is more common in individuals with sickle cell disease.

842. Thayer Martin media is used to grow Neisseria Gonorrhea

843. TZanck media using Geimsa stains is used for herpes simplex

844. Weil Felix reaction is a test for antibodies to Rickettsia organisms such as rickettsia ricketssi that cause rocky mountain spotted fever

845. Ziehl-Neelsen stain is used to test for acid-fast Mycobacterium

846. Charcot's triad consists of fever, jaundice, and right upper quadrant pain indicating acute cholangitis/cholecystitis.

847. It may be complicated by hypotension, confusion, and infection. Infection may be caused by Pseudomonas aeruginosa for which aztreonam is a good antibiotic.

848. Contaminated food with Clostridium botulinum can cause botulism. The baby may be constipated and grow flaccid and weak (floppy baby)

849. Escherichia coli O157: H7 is found in contaminated undercooked beef and can cause the Hemolytic Uremic Syndrome and can be fatal. The endotoxin causes endothelial injury, hemolysis, platelet aggregation and acute renal injury.

850. Rota virus is found infecting nurseries and can cause gastroenteritis

851. Shigella can cause bloody diarrhea and infrequently can cause Hemolytic uremic syndrome.

852. Vibrio cholera is a comma-shaped organism causing massive amounts of diarrhea and can cause death in 50 percent of untreated people due to severe dehydration. Cholera is transmitted through the fecal oral route via contaminated water.

853. Assertive oral rehydration therapy is key to survival in patients with cholera. The oral rehydration mixture is as follows: Water mixed with glucose, NaCl (table salt),

nahco3 Sodium bicarbonate (baking powder), and k (potassium).

854. The SRY gene on the Y chromosome

Induces the development of testes and the male phenotype (appearance)

855. Development of male external genitalia is controlled by DHT.

856. DHT also controls the development of the prostate from the urogenital sinus

857. Prostate cancer is the most common cancer in males, slow growing

858. Prostate cancer is more frequent in African American males

859. Risk factors are family history, race, and smoking

860. Screening test for prostate cancer is PSA or the prostate-specific antigen

861. Frequently metastasizes to the spine, liver and lungs-

862. Seminomas are the most common testicular cancers in young men (age 15 to 35)

863. Characterized by large cells in lobules and a "fried egg" appearance

864. Reineke crystals are seen with Leydig cell tumors

865. Yolk cell tumors may have structures resembling glomeruli

866. Endometriosis-associated with infertility and epithelial ovarian cancer

867. Pelvic inflammatory disease leads to increased risk for ectopic pregnancy

868. Placenta Previa presents as painless vaginal bleeding after 20 weeks of pregnancy

869. History of prior abortion or curettage of the uterine wall can be a risk factor. Prior c section and multiple prior pregnancies are also a risk factor for placenta previa.

870. History of prior ectopic pregnancy increases risk for future ectopic pregnancies

871. Use of assisted reproductive technologies is associated with multiple embryos i.e. twins, triplets

872. In an older male, trouble initiating a stream and postvoidal dribbling are signs of benign prostatic hypertrophy (BPH) until proven otherwise

873. A Foley catheter can help relieve the acute obstruction.

874. Alpha blockers also help with this problem for the long term

875. Hydatidiform mole (complete mole) is caused by an empty egg fertilized by two sperm each contributing an x chromosome leading to 46xx. Both the xx are paternal. There is no fetus, but a trophoblast develops that looks like a cluster of grapes, and the HCG is elevated

876. Partial moles have a contribution from the maternal egg also and may have some fetal parts and a similar grape-like growth.

877. Herpes genital infections are associated with multiple painful lesions and are treated with a 10 day course of acyclovir. Tzanck test reveals multinucleated giant cells with viral inclusion bodies.

878. Chancroid is the other painful genital infection- with single painful sore with exudate at base of ulcer- treated with oral azithromycin.

879. Syphilis sores are painless- treated with Penicillin

880. Oxytocin is produced by paraventricular nucleus of the hypothalamus and is released from the posterior pituitary. It is stored in the nerve terminals before release in what are called Herring bodies

881. Oxytocin is responsible for the dilation of the cervix during labor and contraction of the uterus during labor.

882. A synthetic analog of oxytocin is applied to the cervix is facilitate labor when it is delayed

883. Oxytocin is responsible for the letdown of the milk during breastfeeding.

884. Preeclampsia is characterized by hypertension and proteinuria. Other symptoms include swelling of the face (due to protein loss), headaches, confusion(due to htn), blurred vision (due to htn)

885. Hyperreflexia and thrombocytopenia may be noted.

886. HELLP syndrome may occur and indicates a bad prognosis for the mother and child

887. HELLP syndrome stands for Hemolysis, Elevated liver enzymes, and Low Platelet count (thrombocytopenia mentioned earlier)

888. If seizures occur- it is termed eclampsia

889. Eclampsia is a medical emergency and needs very careful management.

890. Delivery of the baby is curative.

891. Magnesium is given to prevent seizures. Dilantin and diazepam can also be given.

892. Emergency C-Section is the definitive treatment.

893. Fluoroquinolone antibiotics (ciprofloxacin, ofloxacin, norfloxacin) work well for most diarrheal pathogens that cause traveler's diarrhea such as E Coli, Campylobacter Jejuni, Shigellosis, ETEC

894. Enterotoxigenic Escherichia coli (ETEC) is a type of Escherichia coli and the leading bacterial cause of diarrhea in the developing world, as well as the most common cause of travelers' diarrhea

895. Salpingitis is inflammation of the fallopian tubes

896. Chlamydia is the most common cause of sexually transmitted disease.

ACID BASE PHYSIOLOGY

897. A person who is vomiting or having his stomach suctioned will be losing hcl.

So he will have hypochloremic, and hypokalemic metabolic alkalosis -profile. The hypokalemia goes with it. Summary: Low K, Low Cl, increased Ph (alkalosis) due to loss of acid (H+)

Treatment of above is replacement of fluids with normal saline and supplementation of K

Because of the loss of acid and resultant metabolic alkalosis, the kidneys try to excrete the bicarbonate as sodium bicarbonate.

The sodium is reabsorbed, and K and H ions are excreted. That is why you have the low potassium. The loss of H ions is not good, but that is how it works. The resultant urine is said to be paradoxically acidic

898. Partial pressures of Co2 or PaCo2 are more reliable measures of alveolar ventilation than arterial oxygen partial pressures.

The alveolar partial pressures are expressed with a capital A

For example PACO2.

The normal arterial partial pressure of $PaCO_2$ is about 40 mm Hg.

899. Volume loss increases bicarbonate reabsorption by the kidneys.

900. Hypokalemia increases with reabsorption of bicarbonate

901. During blood transfusions, the citrate in the banked blood may lead chelation of calcium leading to low Ca levels, leading to tetany symptoms, Chvostek's sign (tapping on the angle of the jaw causes facial muscles to twitch or contract)

902. Chvostek's sign is the twitching of the facial muscles in response to tapping over the area of the facial nerve. Trousseau's sign is carpopedal spasm caused by inflating the blood-pressure cuff to a level above systolic pressure for 3 minutes.

Treatment is with iv calcium

903. Low calcium levels can lead to prolongation of Qtc

904. Loss of fluids from small intestine (duodenum, jejunum, ileum) are best replaced by Ringer lactate.

905. Ringer's lactate solution is very often used for fluid resuscitation after a blood loss due to trauma, surgery, or a burn injury.[citation needed] Ringer's lactate solution is used because the by-products of lactate

metabolism in the liver counteract acidosis, which is a chemical imbalance that occurs with acute fluid loss or renal failure.

Lactated Ringer's is composed of sodium chloride 6 g/L, sodium lactate 3.1 g/L, potassium chloride 0.3 g/L, and calcium chloride 0.2 g/L.

---

906. Saliva, gastric juice, right colon have high K, low Na content

---

907. The body tries to keep Ph stable with buffers, lungs-respiration, kidneys

908. Important intracellular buffers are proteins and phosphates

909. The bicarbonate-carbonic acid system is the primary extracellular buffer mechanism mediated by the lungs and the kidneys.

---

910. The acids such as lactic acid, pyruvic acid combine with sodium bicarbonate to form sodium salt and carbonic acid which then degrades to h2o and co2. The Co2 is blown off by the lungs. During acidotic states such ad diabetic ketoacidosis, the respiration is therefore increased to blow off the generated co2.

911. Acids + NaHco3 (Sodium bicarbonate)→NaCl + H2Co3 (carbonic acid)-> H2o+ Co2 (blown out by lungs)

912. The kidneys also excrete or retain bicarbonate or H ions to moderate the Ph towards normal.

913. Metabolic Acidosis occurs through the increase of acids such as when lactic acidosis occurs in times of low oxygen or low perfusion, diabetes, **or** loss of bicarbonates such due to diarrhea, bowel fistula or renal dysfunction.

914. Initial compensation for metabolic acidosis is respiratory (hyperventilation), later kidneys help

915. Kidneys help reduce metabolic acidosis by excreting acidic salts and retaining bicarbonate.

916. The commonest cause of acidosis in surgical patients is lactic acidosis due to decreased perfusion and anaerobic metabolism.

917. In metabolic acidosis, the numerator (the upper part) of the Henderson Hasselback equation is affected.

918. Volume replacement with balanced solutions or blood should be the primary therapy for metabolic acidosis in surgery due to blood loss. Ventilation is also important.

919. Overcorrection of metabolic acidosis with aggressive bicarbonate therapy should be avoided.

920. The initial dose of bicarbonate should not exceed 50 ml of 7.5% solution.

METABOLIC ALKALOSIS

This is due to loss of acids such as in prolonged vomiting or gastric suctioning or loss of bicarbonate from diarrhea.

921. Hypokalemia should be monitored for and corrected when present.

---

922. RESPIRATORY ACIDOSIS

Is caused by decreased alveolar ventilation and retention of CO_2.

Treatment is to increase respiration by reversal of respiratory depression, removal of the respiratory obstruction.

For chronic respiratory problems and distress, the kidneys counter by increasing bicarbonate retention in the kidneys.

---

923. For respiratory depression due to opiates, naloxone (Narcan) is the antidote of choice. It is short acting however so some may have to be added in the drip or sequential IM narcan shots have to be given.

924. Naltrexone is the oral long acting opiate antagonist

925. For someone who is opiate dependent, opiate withdrawal symptoms may be precipitated.

Withdrawal symptoms from opiates are runny nose, diarrhea, muscle pain, yawning

926. In pregnant women, opiate withdrawal may lead to premature labor.

927. For benzodiazepines such as lorazepam, diazepam overdose, flumazenil (Brand name Romazicon) is the antidote. Benzo overdose can become lethal when other sedating agents are on board such as alcohol, barbiturates or other CNS depressant meds

928. It is important to Know the concepts of mean (average), the mode (most frequent), and the median (the middle value)

929. Most biological values are distributed along a normal curve

It is the bell shaped curve

930. Standard deviation is a measure of the spread of the data set.

It is the average deviation around the mean value of a data set. In a normal bell curve, two standard deviations cover 95% of the data of the data distribution.

If the data falls outside of the 95% spread (or 2SD), it is felt to be a statistically significant finding.

931. Incidence is the number of new cases in a time period

932. Prevalence is the total number of cases at any one point in time.

933. Duration of illness determines prevalence.

If the illness lasts only a brief period like a common cold, then its incidence may be high for the winter months but total prevalence might be low because it goes away.

Diabetes on the other hand has a low incidence but once diagnosed, it tends to persist so that the prevalence can be high and can increase if the new cases keep occurring.

934. Positive Predictive Value – The likelihood that a positive test is truly positive

935. Negative Predictive Value- The likelihood that a negative test is truly negative.

936. Acrodermatitis Enteropathica is an autosomal recessive disease of children associated with the malabsorption of zinc. This interferes with granulation tissue formation in the process of wound healing.

937. Diagnosis is confirmed by the presence of low zinc levels below hundred milligrams per deciliter.

938. SIADH is associated with normovolemic hyponatremia

939. In polydipsia, hypervolemia would be noted along with hyponatremia.

940. Acute respiratory distress syndrome or ARDS is associated with bilateral interstitial infiltrates before clinical symptoms appear.

941. The best evidence for acute tubular necrosis is the presence of renal tubular cells and muddy brown casts in the urine sediment.

942. An IVP (Intravenous pyelography) is contraindicated in the presence of acute renal failure due to the risk of further precipitation of the dye due to low renal perfusion.

943. Acute suppurative thyroiditis is rare and is caused by an acute bacterial infection.

   (Suppurative means associated with pus.)

944. Exogenous steroid administration is the most common cause of adrenal insufficiency.

945. In adrenal insufficiency, the serum sodum is low and potassium in the serum is elevated. Normally the aldosterone retains the sodium and excretes the potassium. To repeat, In a state of adrenal insufficiency, sodium retention is decreased leading to hyponatremia and there is an associated rise of potassium.

946. A patient with partial albinism and a bleeding disorder probably has dense granule deficiency disease. The platelets are dysfunctional.

947. In alcoholism, there is an accumulation of triglycerides within the hepatocytes.

948. In Alzheimer's disease, there is a neuronal loss in the cerebral cortex. It is also associated with neurofibrillary tangles. The hippocampus is affected more.

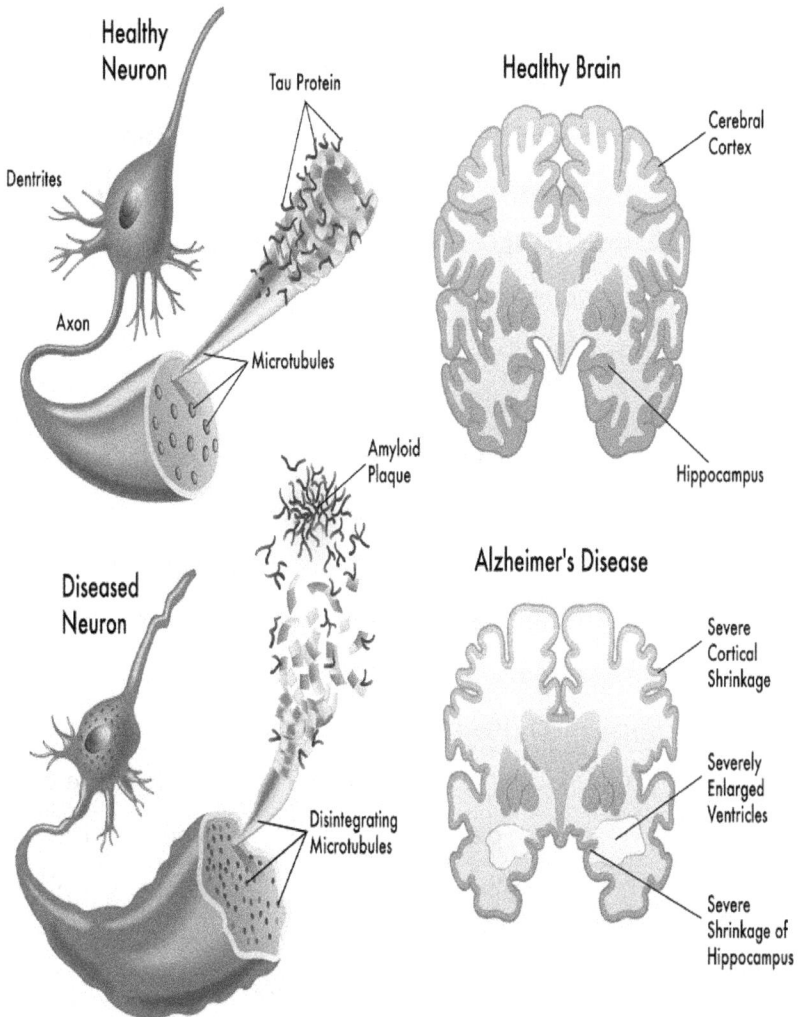

949. Amourosis Fugax is a transient stroke of the eye and is caused by an occlusion of the retinal artery by emboli. Seen on the fundoscopic exam as Hollenhorst plaques.

950. The blindness is unilateral to the side of the retinal artery and is described as a window shade being pulled over that eye. It may last minutes to a few hours.

951. Amniotic fluid embolization can lead to DIC (Disseminated intravascular coagulation)

952. The IgG antibodies are involved in the type I allergic reactions also called anaphylaxis.

953. Anaplastic thyroid cancer has the lowest incidence but the most aggressive course.

954. The antiphospholipid syndrome is marked by the presence of antiphospholipid antibodies, a prolonged PTT, thrombosis, a positive VDRL and a history of spontaneous abortions.

955. A person with prolonged a PTT and thrombosis most likely has the antiphospholipid antibody syndrome.

956. Ascites results from decreased oncotic pressure caused by a decrease in levels of albumin. The decreased albumin is due to decreased production of albumin by the liver because of declining function caused by cirrhosis caused by the alcoholism or other causes.

957. Renal artery stenosis can cause secondary hypertension. The mechanism of the hypertension is due to the stimulation of the renin-angiotensin system activated by the decreased perfusion in that kidney.

958. The kidney affected by renal artery stenosis may shrink in size or atrophy while the opposite side kidney may have compensatory hypertrophy.

959. Atypical ductal hyperplasia may be associated with an increased risk for malignancy. A mild atypical ductal hyperplasia involves 3 to 4 cell layers above the basement membrane and him moderate degree of hyperplasia involves five or more cell layers above the basement membrane.

960. Basal cell carcinoma: the aggressive behavior of this cancer when it occurs is mediated by collagenase production.

961. Nevus sebaceous of Jadasshohn is associated with basal cell carcinoma. It can present as a alopecic leathery patch on the scalp.

962. Bell's palsy is most commonly associated with infection by herpes simplex virus

963. Marfan's syndrome- proteins affected are fibrillin, elastin, mutation is on Chromosome 15 called FBNI mutation

964. They are pushing the use of statins on the test for even mildly elevated cholesterol, so go with it.

965. Familial hypocalciuric syndrome is a rare genetic cause of hypercalcemia. Not enough calcium is excreted in urine so the plasma ca level is elevated.

966. Parathyroid adenoma is the usual suspect in the cause of hypercalcemia.

967. Milk alkali syndrome is elevated calcium due to excessive intake of calcium. Can occur if someone takes a lot of antacid such as calcium hydroxide, or is trying to treat osteoporosis with Ca supplements.

968. Someone with cirrhosis and ascites can develop spontaneous peritonitis due to an infection that can present as abdominal pain. Fever may not be present; antibiotic cefotaxime recommended until culture results available.

969. Tourette's disorder can present with vocal and motor tics and is not a seizure disorder. Treatment is dopamine blocker such as pimozide or haloperidol.

970. Ventriculoseptal defect is the most common congenital heart defect. Most close soon after birth. May be associated with Down's syndrome.

971. Alcohol withdrawal may present as confusion, elevated vitals within 24 to 48 hours of last drink. Keep this differential high in someone with a history of alcoholism disclosed or undisclosed. Surgical patients in post-operative care may run into an alcohol withdrawal problem when they have not disclosed their daily drinking habit.

972. Acidosis can cause the shift to the right of the oxygen dissociation curve.

973. Genital Herpes- painful shallow ulcers on genitalia surface, fever, headache, muscle pain associated

974. Gonorrhea associated with purulent discharge

975. Intracellular diplococci cause Neisseria gonorrhea cause gonorrhea.

976. In psychiatric patients acute neck stiffness is caused by antipsychotics such as haloperidol, fluphenazine-treatment is with benztropine 2 mgs IM or PO, diphenhydramine (Benadryl) 50 mgs IM or PO can also be used.

977. Akathisia is a sense of restlessness caused by antipsychotics – treatment is with benztropine and or beta blockers such as propranolol

978. Tardive Dyskinesia is a syndrome of involuntary movements associated with the long-term use of antipsychotics.

979. Pulmonary hypertension is when the pulmonary artery pressure is greater than the 70% of the systemic pressure. May present as dyspnea in a pregnant young mother. Risk to mother is significant if present, may be a reason for elective medical termination of pregnancy MTP or abortion.

980. Trick Question: A Brain biopsy is the <u>most accurate test to confirm </u>a brain tumor. A MRI or CT scan may ordered as an initial screen in that preferential order.

981. HIV drug zidovidine causes mitochondrial changes in cells.

982. HIV, Simvastatin, Alcohol, cocaine abuse can cause myositis.

983. Takayasu arteritis is found in young Asian females is an arteritis that can cause low blood pressure, muscle pains. Wt loss is common

984. Acute tubular necrosis is result of volume loss. Rise in blood urea nitrogen (azotemia), Cr, Muddy brown epithelial casts and granular casts found in urine, proteinuria

985. humpy lumpy deposits in acute glomerulonephritis. Type III reaction.

986. Interstitial nephritis is reaction around tubules caused by drugs, infection. Eosinophilia may occur.

987. Hypothyroidism associated with wt gain, menstrual irregularities, galactorrhea, sensitivity to cold, constipation, dry skin, slowed tendon reflexes

988. For influenza, amantadine and zanamivir are helpful if indicated in the first 48 hours of the onset of symptoms.

989. ACE inhibitors such as Lisinopril or ARB's such as losartan are first line agents for many individuals with hypertension due to the protective effect provided to the kidneys for nephropathy related to hypertension.

990. ARB's have the advantage of not causing the side effect of cough that can occur with some ACE inhibitors.

991. Doxazosin is an smooth muscle relaxer (selective alpha 1 blocker) that is used for htn in patients that also have prostatic hypertrophy (BPH) as it helps both the conditions. Dizziness upon arising is a risk with alpha blockers. This is called orthostatic hypotension (blood pools in the lower legs upon arising leading to decrease in blood pressure and dizziness. With time, body makes adjustments)

992. Colonoscopy is recommended for all persons after 50 as screening for CA colon and then every 10 years if no polyps.

993. A person is deemed competent and has the right to refuse medication and care. Only a court of law can deem a patient to be incompetent and may appoint a conservator.

994. Pain in the flank, costovertebral tenderness and fever can have a high chance of being acute pyelonephritis. Get UA, culture, treat as indicated by sensitivity.

995. Brief psychotic disorder lasts from a day to <u>less than a month</u> . It is is induced in some people by acute stressors.

996. A child with hematuria, deafness, eye problems and family member with similar problems may have Alport's syndrome – x linked recessive.

997. In Wilm's tumor caused by chromosome 11 disorder, children age 2-4 years of age present with a flank mass that may be palpable. Hematuria may also be be present.

998. Wilms tumor is sometimes associated with aniridia, genitourinary symptoms and retardation. This is called the WAGRS complex.

999. C-11 hydroxylase deficiency can present as precocious early puberty, hypertension and aggressive behaviors due to high testosterone levels from stimulation of adrenal glands .

1000. C21 hydroxylase also leads to increased testosterone levels, and low cortisol and aldosterone levels. It leads to low blood pressure due to low aldosterone.

1001. 17 hydroxylase deficiency leads to delayed puberty.

1002. 22q11 syndrome (DiGeorge Syndrome) associated with Tetralogy of Fallot and persistent truncus arteriosus.

1003. Infants of Diabetic mother have a higher risk for transposition of great vessels

1004. Fungal infection of toes causes discoloration, hyphae seen under microscope

1005. Topical radiation therapy is the treatment of choice for first stage vaginal cancer.

1006. More infiltrative vaginal cancer may need surgery and radiation. Chemotherapy is used after surgery as well. Hormonal treatment is not indicated.

1007. The most common age of onset of eczema is 1-2 years of age. Skin is dry and scaly.

1008. Seborrheic dermatitis, dandruff can affect immunocompromised individuals more often

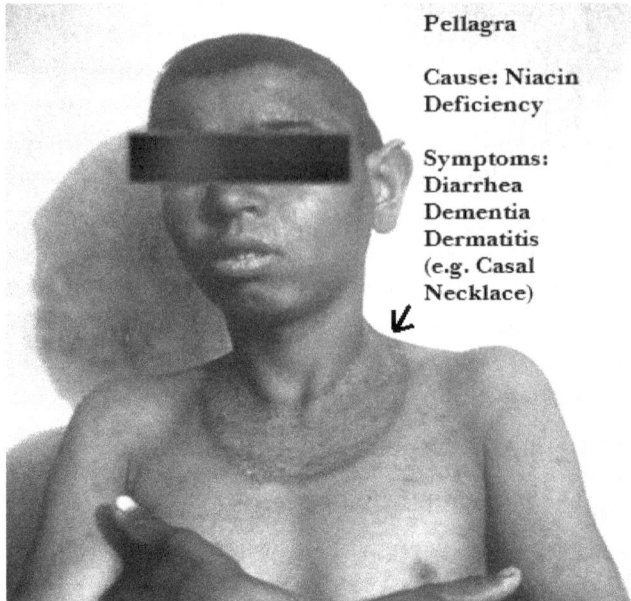

Pellagra

Cause: Niacin Deficiency

Symptoms:
Diarrhea
Dementia
Dermatitis
(e.g. Casal Necklace)

1009.
Credit: CDC http://phil.cdc.gov/phil/details.asp

1010. Vitamin A deficiency is associated with night blindness.

1011. Vitamin C deficiency causes scurvy

1012. Vit D deficiency causes rickets in children and osteomalacia in adults.

1013. Deficiency of folic acid in pregnant mothers can cause neural tube defects in the infant.

1014. Choriocarcinoma is a cancer of the placenta. HCG is elevated. May spread to lungs. Symptoms may include abnormal vaginal bleeding after the recent birth of a child.

1015. Testicular torsion may present with acute abdominal pain and is a surgical emergency.

1016. N acetyl cysteine is the treatment of choice for an overdose of acetaminophen.

1017. Pyridoxine is drug of choice for INH poisoning

1018. Fomepizole is drug of choice for methanol poisoning or ethylene glycol poisoning.

1019. Calcium gluconate for hydrofluoric acid toxicity

1020. Next step is often different from the diagnostic step, read the question carefully.

1021. For an elderly person who is found wandering in the neighborhood in a confused state and there are no medical problems: The next step would be to do a mini mental status exam.

1022. Alexia is the loss of ability to read. It is related to strokes in the area of the posterior cerebral artery.

1023. Apraxia is the loss of ability to do simple tasks. Posterior parietal cortex involved.

1024. Aphasia is result of damage to temporal speech area. Anterior damage associated with Broca's aphasia- lack of ability to speak

Wernicke's aphasia is due to damage to posterior temporal area. Person can speak but cannot understand spoken speech

1025. Agnosia is the inability to recognize common objects- due to damage to occipitotemporal border area.

1026. Some jaundice in new born due to elevated unconjugated bilirubin may be normal. Light therapy is helpful.

1027. Aminoglycosides are gentamycin, streptomycin, amikacin, tobramycin

1028. Sideeffects of Aminoglycosides can be remembered with phrase : NO NEED OF TOXINS

Stands for : Nephrotoxicity, Neuromuscular blockade, Ototoxicity, and Teratogen

1029. Parathyroid adenoma is the usual suspect in the cause of hypercalcemia.

1030. For influenza, amantadine and zanamivir are helpful if indicated in the first 48 hours of the onset of symptoms.

1031. ACE inhibitors such as Lisinopril or ARB's such as losartan are first line agents for many individuals with hypertension due to the protective effect provided to the kidneys for nephropathy related to hypertension.

1032. ARB's have the advantage of not causing the side effect of cough that can occur with some ACE inhibitors.

1033. Doxazosin is an smooth muscle relaxer (selective alpha 1 blocker) that is used for htn in patients that also have prostatic hypertrophy (BPH) as it helps both the conditions. Dizziness upon arising is a risk with alpha blockers. This is called orthostatic hypotension (blood pools in the lower legs upon arising leading to decrease in blood pressure and dizziness. With time, body makes adjustments)

1034. Hydralazine is also a smooth muscle blocker but is not used much due to side effect of causing SLE like syndrome.

1035. Mycosis Fungoides

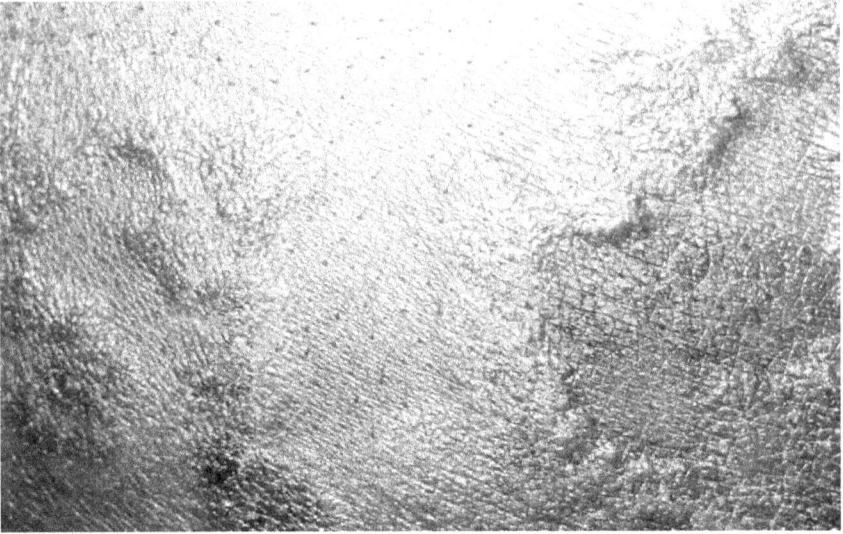

CDC/ Renelle Woodall

http://phil.cdc.gov/phil/details.asp

Mycosis fungoides depicted above is not a fungal infection. It is a form of T cell Non-Hodgkin's lymphoma with cutaneous manifestations. It is also known as Alibert-Bazin syndrome.

1099   Zika Virus - A RNA Flavivirus

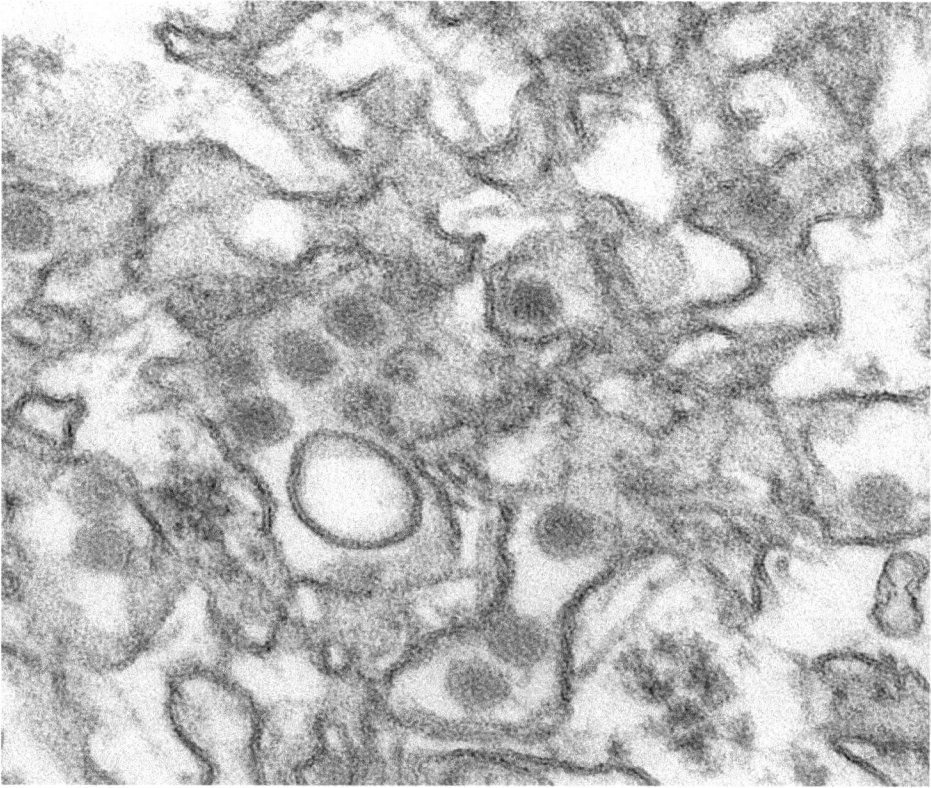

CDC/ Cynthia Goldsmith

In the above picture, the virus particles are colored red. It is spread by the Aedes mosquito- the same mosquito that transmits yellow fever. The syndrome is marked by the following symptoms that last a few days to a week- fever, joint pain, conjunctivitis (red eyes). The virus can also be transmitted sexually if one of the partner is infected. If a woman contracts this illness during her pregnancy, it may lead to developmental delays in the child including microcephaly. Not all infants are affected.

1036. Inclusion Conjunctivitis caused by Chlamydia Trachomatis

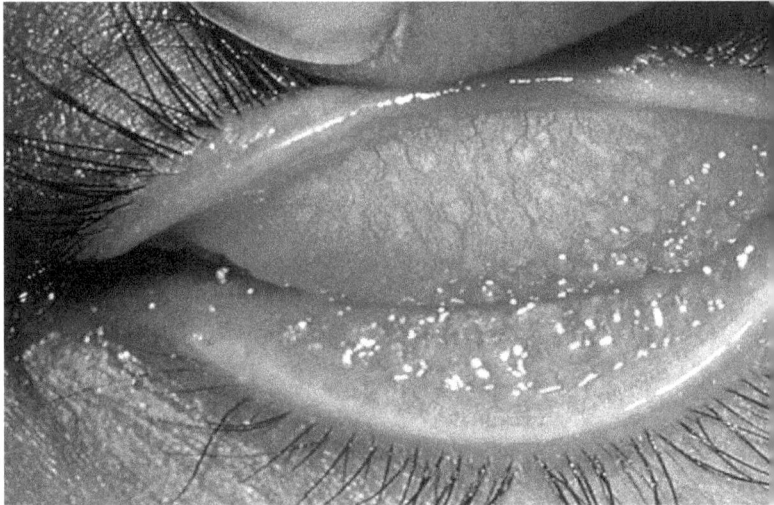

CDC/ Susan Lindsley   Inclusion Conjunctivitis caused by Chlamydia Trachomatis

1037. Inclusion conjunctivitis shown above is caused by Chlamydia trachomatis Serovar Ab, B, B or C. It can cause trachoma and is leading cause of blindness. It is also the most frequent cause of STD in the United States.

1038. The Chlaymdia trachomatis is an obligate intracellular parasite and has three antigenic strains called biovars.

1039. Serovars Ab B Ba and C – cause infection of the eye depicted above, and trachoma that can lead to blindness.

1040. Serovars D- K - causes STD's- pelvic inflammatory disease, urethritis, salpingitis which lead to impaired fertility or ectopic pregnancy in women. These strains have also been linked to neonatal pneumonia and neonatal conjunctivitis.

1041. Servars L1, L2, L3 causes the distinct STD Lymphgranuloma venereum.

1042. Some Chlamydia have an extrachromosomal DNA called plasmid. The chlamydia can share genetic information and this can lead to the formation of new strains.

1043. A CD4 T lymphocyte count of less than 200 suggests the presence of AIDS.

1044. Decreased T Cells are seen DiGeorge syndrome because of the absence of the thymus.

1045. In Bruton X linked agammaglobulunemia there is a deficit in humoral (antibody) immunity due to a failure of B lymphocyte maturation. The child is vulnerable to pyogenic infections. The child may be protected for the first few months due to the passive immunity received from the mother's igG recived through the placenta. In this syndrome, the tonsils, adenoids are absent.

1046. Selective IgA deficiency is the most common inherited immunodeficiency in European populations.

If such a person receives blood or plasma, they may mount an antigenic response to the IgA that he or she does not have naturally in their own blood. This may come as a surprise as the blood groups have been matched prior to the transfusion. This reaction however is to the IgA antibody and not to the person's blood group.

1047. Type II reaction occurs in the mother that is Rh-, and has Rh+ baby. This leads to lysis of red blood cells and leads to the condition called erythroblastosis fetalis. The condition poses a grave danger to the viability of the pregnancy.

1048. Some other Type II reactions are Rheumatic Fever, Grave's Disease, and Goodpasture Syndrome.

1049. Type III reactions are SLE, Glomerulonephritis, Polyarteritis Nodosa

1050. Type IV reactions are PPD skin test, transplant rejection, and contact dermatitis.

1051. Redman Syndrome is an anaphylactic reaction is due to rapid infusion with vancomycin. Can be prevented by slower infusion and pretreatment with an antihistamine.

1052. In microscopic polyangiitis, there are antibodies against enzymes myeloperoxidase. It stains in a perinuclear pattern called P-ANCA (Perinuclear antineutrophil cytoplasmic antibody)

1053. In Wegner's granulomatosis, the antibody is to proteinase 3 called C-ANCA (cytoplasmic antineutrophil cytoplasmic antibody).

www.ingramcontent.com/pod-product-compliance
Lightning Source LLC
Chambersburg PA
CBHW060608200326
41521CB00007B/703